KU-496-914

DIAGNOSIS OF
BREAST DISEASE

Imaging, Clinical Features and Pathology

DIAGNOSIS OF BREAST DISEASE

Imaging, Clinical Features and Pathology

Edited by

C.A. PARSONS

Consultant Radiologist,
Royal Marsden Hospital,
London and Sutton

LONDON

CHAPMAN AND HALL

First published 1983
by Chapman and Hall Ltd,
11 New Fetter Lane, London EC4P 4EE
© *1983 Chapman and Hall Ltd*

Typeset by Servis Filmsetting Ltd
and printed in Great Britain at the
University Press, Cambridge

ISBN 0 412 22130 6

All rights reserved. No part of
this book may be reprinted, or reproduced
or utilized in any form or by any electronic,
mechanical or other means, now known or hereafter
invented, including photocopying and recording,
or in any information storage or retrieval
system, without permission in writing
from the publisher

British Library Cataloguing in Publication Data

Diagnosis of breast disease.
1. Breast – Diseases
I. Parsons, C.A.
618.1′9075   RG493

ISBN 0-412-22130-6

CONTENTS

List of Contributors   *page* vii

Preface   ix

1. **Principles of breast pathology**   I
    R. Millis

2. **Clinical features of breast disease**   26
    J.A. McKinna

3. **Mammographic technique**   54
    O. Wilson

4. **Physics of mammography**   76
    D.R. Dance and R. Davis

5. **Mammographic features of benign disease**   101
    C.A. Parsons

6. **Mammographic features of malignancy**   142
    C.A. Parsons

7. **Practical diagnostic procedures**   192
    C.A. Parsons and J.A. McKinna

8. **Cytological investigation**   203
    P.A. Trott

9. **Thermography of the female breast**   214
    C.H. Jones

10.   **Ultrasound in breast diagnosis**   235
       T.S. Reeve, J. Jellins, G. Kossoff and
       B.H. Barraclough

11.   **Diagnosis in clinical practice**   248
       J.A. McKinna and J. Davey

       Bibliography   264

       Index   279

LIST OF CONTRIBUTORS

B.H. BARRACLOUGH, MB, BS, FRACS
Visiting Surgeon, The Westmead Centre, Westmead, New South Wales, Australia. Clinical Consultant, Ultrasonics Institute, Sydney, Australia.

D.R. DANCE, MA, PhD
Principal Physicist, The Royal Marsden Hospital, London.

JANE B. DAVEY, MB, BS
Medical Officer in Charge, Early Diagnostic Unit, The Royal Marsden Hospital, London.

R. DAVIS, FIST
Senior Research Assistant, Physics Department, Institute of Cancer Research and The Royal Marsden Hospital, London.

J. JELLINS, BSc, BE, MAC, PSM
Head of Ultrasonic Imaging Section, Ultrasonics Institute, Sydney, Australia. Consultant in Clinical Ultrasound, The Royal North Shore Hospital, St. Leonards, New South Wales, Australia.

C.H. JONES, BSc, PhD, FInstP
Senior Lecturer, Institute of Cancer Research and The Royal Marsden Hospital, London.

G. KOSSOFF, BSc, ME, FAIUM
Director, Ultrasonics Institute, Sydney, Australia. Consultant in Clinical Ultrasound, The Royal North Shore Hospital, St. Leonards, New South Wales, Australia.

A.J. McKINNA, FRCS
Consultant Surgeon, The Royal Marsden Hospital, London.

ROSEMARY R. MILLIS, MB, BS, MRCPath
Consultant Pathologist, Guy's Health District and the Imperial
Cancer Research Fund Breast Cancer Unit, Guy's Hospital,
London. Honorary Research Consultant, The Breast Unit, The
Royal Marsden Hospital, London.

C.A. PARSONS, MB, BS, FRCS, FRCR
Consultant Radiologist, The Royal Marsden Hospital, London.

T.S. REEVE, CBE, MB, BS, FACS, FRACS
Professor, Department of Surgery, University of Sydney, The
North Shore Hospital, St. Leonards, New South Wales, Australia.

P.A. TROTT, MB, BChir(Cantab), MRCPath
Consultant Pathologist, The Royal Marsden Hospital, London.

OLIVIA WILSON
Superintendent Radiographer, Early Diagnostic Unit, The Royal
Marsden Hospital, London.

PREFACE

The successful diagnosis of breast disease relies upon the close collaboration of a team of specialists comprising of clinicians, radiologists, radiographers, cytologists and histologists. Although each member of the team has his own expertise, the overall contribution he can make will be greatly enhanced by possessing at least a basic understanding of the capabilities and failings of the other specialities. The radiologist needs to know a good deal of breast pathology and to understand the implications of particular clinical features if he is to provide sound advice when mammographic features are atypical. Similarly, the surgeon who cannot accurately interpret mammograms will waste a lot of effort heading down the wrong diagnostic pathway, losing patient confidence as he goes. Review meetings at which clinical, cytological and mammographic features are compared with a definitive histological diagnosis provides an excellent means for developing this understanding, and much of the material in this text derives from such case discussions. It is very difficult for an individual working in isolation to accumulate the knowledge and experience, from outside his own speciality, which he needs to develop the best approach to the various clinical problems which arise. The multi-disciplinary format of this book should be particularly useful for those who are in this situation.

After physical examination, mammography has become the most important additional diagnostic procedure in breast disease. To obtain images of high quality, a clear understanding of the physical principles of mammography is required and, when available, a medical physicist's co-operation should be sought to establish the imaging system, determine the actual radiation dose to the patient and institute methods to keep this as low as possible without impairing optimum image quality. The mammographic features of breast pathology are the same whether they are recorded on film or by xerography, and can be learned from either system. This book is illustrated with xerographic images, though users of film should find little difficulty in comparing them with the output of their own departments. Although familiarity with a particular system does, of course, enable the radiologist to recognize abnormalities more quickly in that format, the extensive illustrations given in Chapters 5 and 6 should form useful reference material for any mammographer, whether he uses film or xerography.

Diagnostic methods are in constant evolution. New procedures which can be shown to be accurate and reliable gradually become established, replacing those of lesser value. The most useful new technique is undoubtedly fine-needle aspiration cytology, which in experienced hands provides an extremely high true positive rate of diagnosis, and yet relies heavily on the clinician to sample the appropriate area properly. The success of the technique is indicated by the increasing number of pathologists anxious to acquire the necessary experience. Ultrasound has not yet reached this stage of acceptance but of all the new imaging methods it is the most interesting, particularly where it is used to answer a specific question which arises during clinical and mammographic examination. Thermography is perhaps not so widely used as it used to be and certainly has a very different role. Like most diagnostic modalities, thermography is most valuable in the hands of those who are able to devote time and extreme care to the evaluation of a relatively small number of patients, particularly if a time series of patients' thermal patterns can be collected. By presenting the reader with all of these aspects of current practice it is hoped that this book will help him to select those modalities which will serve him and his patients best.

I am grateful for the co-operation of my colleagues in contributing chapters to this textbook and for their support in day-to-day practice. My thanks are also due to my secretary, Mrs Catherine Greenland, who has so patiently assisted with the manuscript.

Colin Parsons
London

PRINCIPLES OF
BREAST PATHOLOGY

Rosemary Millis

The final diagnosis of breast cancer depends on histological examination. However suspicious the clinical or radiological signs may be, definitive treatment should not be undertaken until the diagnosis has been confirmed by histology.

DIAGNOSTIC PROCEDURES

In the past the most usual form of management of operable breast cancer consisted of frozen section followed, after a positive diagnosis, by immediate mastectomy under the same anaesthetic. Recently, increasing use of a two-stage procedure has been adopted, with diagnostic biopsy followed several days later by definitive surgery. There are advantages and disadvantages to both approaches, and the best method of management varies with different patients in different situations.

Frozen section

The use of the frozen section technique necessitates only one operation and minimizes the time between detection and definitive treatment. Using the modern cryostat, frozen sections are of a very high standard, being only slightly inferior to those prepared from routinely processed tissue in paraffin blocks. Nevertheless the interpretation of frozen sections can be difficult and, whenever possible, some unfrozen tissue should be preserved for the preparation of paraffin sections, since freezing and thawing may result in ice crystal artefacts which can distort the histological picture. Apart from difficulties of interpretation, the frozen section technique is also liable to sampling errors. In the case of a grossly obvious lesion there is usually no problem. However, a very small carcinoma can be missed, particularly if the tissue sample is large, or an occult carcinoma may be present in the tissue surrounding an obvious benign lesion. Furthermore it is important that multiple blocks of tissue containing an *in situ* carcinoma are prepared and multiple sections scrutinised before the possibility of invasion can be excluded. It should always be remembered that a frozen section report is only preliminary and it is often better to forgo frozen section in the absence of a grossly obvious lesion, particularly when the biopsy is performed on the basis of an abnormal mammogram.

Separate biopsy

The two-stage procedure in the management of primary, operable breast cancer also has advantages. Once a positive diagnosis has been made, the patient can be adequately assessed and the extent of the disease fully evaluated before major surgery is undertaken. The procedure allows for detailed microscopic evaluation of the tumour, which may have some bearing on the surgical treatment. It also allows the clinician to discuss fully with the patient the options for treatment when they both know the exact diagnosis. It eliminates the need for patients to undergo surgery not knowing how extensive their operation is to be, and avoids the necessity of preparing women for the possibility of major surgery who turn out to have a benign lesion. In addition, frozen section inevitably causes delay in the operating theatre, so that dispensing with this procedure permits better planning of operating time.

Biopsy techniques

The initial diagnosis of breast cancer can be made by open biopsy, needle biopsy or aspiration cytology. Open biopsy allows for full evaluation of the tumour histology, but usually necessitates hospitalization and general anaesthesia. However, if the lesion is small and superficial, biopsy can be carried out under a local anaesthetic as an out-patient procedure. Needle biopsy can always be done on an out-patient basis, and is relatively quick, simple and cheap in materials and operating time. The use of an out-patient biopsy procedure has the additional advantage of allowing the patient to be at home with her family to support her during this stressful period.

NEEDLE BIOPSY

Various types of needle are in use, but currently the most popular is probably the 'Tru-cut'. This provides a good sample of tissue with little distortion (Fig. 1.1). In most reported series, needle biopsies provided a positive diagnosis in approximately 75% of mammary carcinomas (Roberts et al., 1975; Elston et al., 1978; Fentiman et al., 1980). False positive results are rare, if they occur at all, but false negative biopsies are not uncommon. A negative needle biopsy should always be followed by a planned open biopsy and can never exclude the presence of a carcinoma. In addition, although needle biopsy samples of mammary carcinoma allow for some evaluation of the tumour type, full assessment can only be made when the entire tumour is examined.

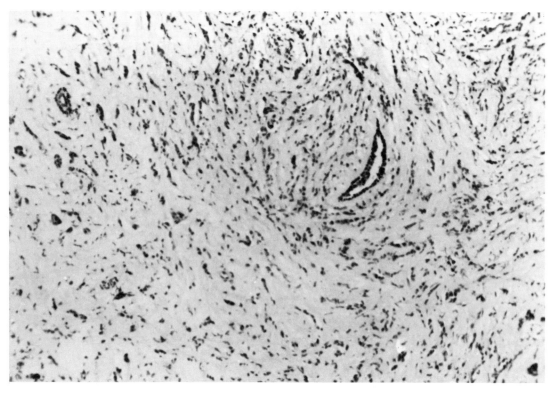

Fig. 1.1   Tru-cut needle biopsy showing a good sample of an infiltrating lobular carcinoma of breast which occupies the full width of the picture. The single file and targetoid pattern of infiltration is well demonstrated. H and E × 100.

The use of aspiration needle biopsy has also grown over recent years and this procedure is discussed fully in Chapter 8.

Gross examination of specimens

Microscopic examination of mammary tissue should always be supplemented by careful gross examination. The two complement each other and accurate histological diagnosis can only be made if the tissue has been adequately and intelligently sampled. Although the initial handling of the tissue depends somewhat on the type of specimen and the clinical and gross findings, examination and dissection should always be carried out in a methodical manner. Blocks of tissue should be taken to include not only those areas which show unusual gross features but also representative samples of all the submitted tissue. If a biopsy is performed because of a lump and a definite lesion is found on gross examination, a preliminary diagnosis can usually be made. The gross appearance of most infiltrating carcinomas is typical, consisting of a firm mass with an irregular outline.

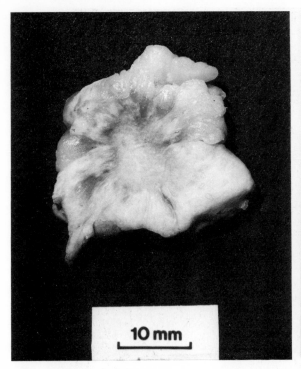

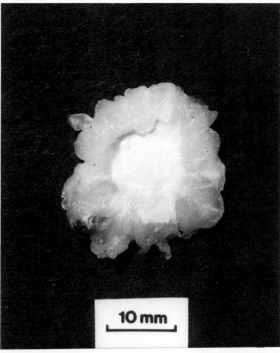

Fig. 1.2   Cut surface of a typical infiltrating duct carcinoma showing the irregular edge, moderately demarcated from the surrounding fibro-fatty breast tissue. The latter is drawn in towards the carcinoma which has a slightly concave surface. Occasional streaks of elastic tissue are seen on the cut surface of the tumour.

Fig. 1.3   Cut surface of an infiltrating duct carcinoma with a partly nodular and partly irregular outline clearly demarcated from the surrounding fatty breast tissue.

Fig. 1.3

Tumours with abundant collagenous stroma have a very characteristic gross and mammographic appearance: tentacles of carcinoma extend into the surrounding tissue and the trabeculae of the adjacent breast are distorted and drawn in towards the tumour mass (Fig. 1.2). The cut surface of most carcinomas feels extremely firm with a very hard edge. The sensation on cutting through the tumour with a knife is typical, the classical comparison with the texture of an unripe pear being very apt; the grittiness is due to the fibrous stroma. Tumours with a very large amount of collagenous stroma and relatively sparse numbers of malignant cells are sometimes called scirrhous. Other carcinomas have a more circumscribed or nodular outline (Fig. 1.3). Usually such tumours contain less stroma or have a dense collagenous centre with a cellular periphery. Some tumours are very cellular containing little stroma and are much softer than the classical scirrhous carcinoma; such growths are sometimes called medullary or encephaloid. They usually have a very smooth round outline, and may be confused both on gross and mammographic appearance with benign lesions. Other less common special varieties of carcinoma may have a similar appearance; these will be described in more detail later.

The outline of a carcinoma may be well- or ill-defined depending upon the nature of the tumour and the surrounding tissue. When the surrounding tissue is fatty and the tumour is fibrous the outline is usually well defined. In a dense breast, particularly if there is less productive

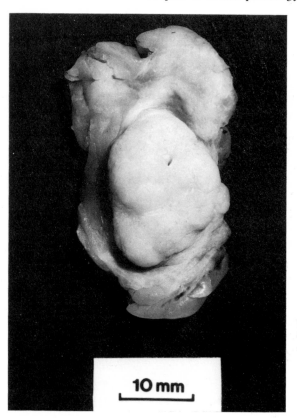

10 mm

Fig. 1.4 Cut surface of a fibroadenoma showing the clearly demarcated rather lobulated neoplasm protruding from the surrounding fibro-fatty breast tissue.

fibrosis within the carcinoma, the tumour edge may not be clear on either gross or mammographic examination as it merges with the surrounding tissue, and the carcinoma can often be better defined by palpation than by vision. The cut surface is usually flush with the adjacent tissue, but may be slightly concave or occasionally bulge, depending on the relative amounts of tumour cells and fibrous stroma. A carcinoma is firmly tethered by infiltration to the surrounding breast tissue, in contrast to a fibroadenoma which is very sharply defined and 'pops out' when cut across as it is 'released' from the compressed surrounding tissue (Fig. 1.4).

The colour of the majority of carcinomas varies from grey to white to pink. The yellowish streaks which are frequently seen on the cut surface, particularly of the firmer tumours, represent elastic tissue within the stroma and not foci of necrosis or calcification as has sometimes been thought.

In situ duct carcinoma is not always discernible on gross examination of the specimen but if a large enough focus is present a mass may be formed. Furthermore, *in situ* duct carcinoma of the comedo type has a particular macroscopic feature which is the extrusion of creamy-yellow cords or 'comedos' of necrotic material from the cut surface of the ducts.

Calcification often occurs within this necrotic material and gives a characteristic mammographic pattern.

When tissue is examined in which there is no obvious gross lesion adequate sampling is important. As mentioned, *in situ* duct carcinoma is frequently not obvious grossly, and *in situ* lobular carcinoma is usually a chance microscopic finding. Some infiltrating carcinomas, in particular infiltrating lobular carcinoma, may also be very diffuse with little productive fibrosis and no well-defined mass. The tumour may thus be difficult to define on gross examination and difficult to see on mammography since the change in density from the surrounding breast tissue is minimal. Even when a definite benign lesion is found on gross examination, the surrounding tissue should always be sampled.

Biopsies on the basis of abnormal mammograms

Tissue that is biopsied on the basis of an abnormal mammogram, particularly in the absence of physical findings, must be studied carefully. It is essential to confirm that the lesional tissue has been removed by comparing radiographs of the biopsy specimen with the pre-operative mammogram. This is especially important when locating calcification. Indeed, specimen radiography may not be so helpful in identifying mammographically suspicious areas that do not contain calcification. Ideally, when the biopsied tissue is removed it should be marked by the surgeon with a radio-opaque label, so that the specimen can be orientated in relation to the radiograph. Additionally, if the suspicious area is found to have been incompletely removed, the geographical area in which excision is incomplete can be identified. The specimen radiograph should be used by the pathologist as a map, when dissecting the tissue, to help localize the area that is under suspicion.

Unless there is an obvious gross lesion it is best to forgo frozen section examination and take multiple blocks for paraffin sections. If the tissue is further radiographed after it has been sliced, blocks can be taken accurately from the areas containing calcification or other mammographic abnormalities. When calcification is the indication for the biopsy its presence must be confirmed microscopically. If not, deeper sections and, if necessary, further tissue should be examined. Radiographs of the spare tissue and the tissue blocks may reveal the site of the calcification. If any doubt remains that the suspicious area on the mammogram has not been removed, a repeat mammogram several months postoperatively should be taken.

Radiography of other specimens

Radiography of specimens removed from the breast is also helpful in biopsy from patients in a high risk category, where the biopsy specimen is extremely large and in cases where preliminary sections have shown *in situ* carcinoma or areas suspicious but not diagnostic of malignancy. However, specimen radiography should never be used to eliminate the need for thorough gross examination and sampling of the biopsy specimen.

Radiographs may be taken in the routine radiography department or in apparatus designed specifically for radiographic examination of tissue within the laboratory. Self-developing polaroid film can be used in such apparatus but some workers claim that it lacks the high degree of resolution necessary for demonstrating fine particles of calcification (Rosen *et al.*, 1974; Gallager, 1975).

Radiography has also been used in the examination of mastectomy specimens to aid mapping of breast lesions when the radiographs can be matched with their gross and microscopical counterparts. Radiography of axillary tissue to aid in the location of lymph nodes may be helpful. However, small or fatty nodes can be missed and differentiation between involved and uninvolved nodes may be possible only if those containing metastases are very large. Careful gross dissection is always necessary.

Gross examination of mastectomy specimens

Just as examination of biopsy specimens should be carried out in a methodical manner, so should the examination of mastectomy specimens. Even though the diagnosis of malignancy has been established, it is nevertheless important to study the remainder of the breast. The axillary lymph nodes should be categorized into three levels so that the extent of axillary involvement can be evaluated. This is facilitated if the surgeon marks the specimen with suitably placed sutures or clips while performing the mastectomy. Low level nodes lie below and lateral to the pectoralis minor muscle, middle level nodes behind the pectoralis minor muscle and high level nodes above the medial edge of the muscle. The nodes should be dissected carefully and as many as possible identified. The number varies considerably from patient to patient and obviously depends to a large degree on the extent of the operation. Some workers find that if the fixed axillary tissue is treated with a solvent such as xylene which clarifies the fat, the nodes are easier to locate, but others find that dissection using careful manual palpation results in a similar yield (Fisher and Slack, 1970). When examining the lymph nodes it should be remembered that not only does the presence or absence of nodal metastases have prognostic significance, but that the number and level of the involved nodes are also important.

Examination of the remainder of the breast tissue should include taking samples of any macroscopic abnormalities as well as routine blocks from the nipple and all four quadrants. Multiple foci of carcinoma may be present and the overall pathology of the remaining breast should be recorded. This is one important approach to the further understanding of breast cancer and its relationship to other pathological changes within the breast.

CLASSIFICATION OF BREAST CARCINOMA

The classification of mammary carcinoma has always been somewhat controversial. This does not mean that pathologists disagree on what should be called malignant or benign: the controversy concerns rather the terminology and histogenesis of the different tumour types. Classifications are based on descriptive morphology or histogenic criteria, the merits and drawbacks of most commonly used systems are well discussed by van Bogaert and Maldague (1978). It is important that a classification should be prognostically useful, easily reproducible and comprehensible. The classification used here is primarily based on histogenic criteria (Table 1.1).

Table 1.1

Classification of mammary carcinoma	Approximate % of different types of carcinoma
In situ carcinoma	
In situ duct carcinoma	5
In situ lobular carcinoma	2
Infiltrating carcinoma	
Infiltrating duct carcinoma	
Without special features	75
With special features	
Medullary carcinoma with lymphoid stroma	3
Mucoid carcinoma	2
Tubular carcinoma	1
Infiltrating lobular carcinoma	10
Rare varieties of mammary carcinoma	1
Papillary carcinoma	
Adenoid cystic carcinoma	
Carcinoma with metaplasia	
Squamous cell carcinoma	
Lipid secreting carcinoma	
Juvenile or secretory carcinoma	
Carcinoma with particular clinical manifestations	
Paget's disease of the nipple	
Inflammatory carcinoma	

There are two major criteria which are used in the majority of classifications of mammary carcinoma: the presence or absence of invasion, and the origin of the tumour from either ducts or lobules. The second criterion was at first thought to be based on the anatomic unit of origin of malignant cells, but the work of Wellings *et al.* (1975) suggests that most carcinomas of all types arise from the same region of the breast, namely the terminal duct lobular unit. This includes the ductule or terminal duct and the blunt ending portions of the mammary duct system, known as terminal ductules, acini or alveoli which collectively form the lobule. Although it was originally thought that all lobular carcinomas arose from the lobular system and ductal carcinomas from the more proximal ducts there is probably considerable overlap and the division is based more on structural and cytological differences than on the anatomic site of origin. The great majority of carcinomas are of the ductal type and further categorization of ductal carcinomas is based on morphological patterns seen macroscopically and microscopically. Usually a combination of features is used in defining the different types of tumour. When selecting tissue blocks from a carcinoma for histological examination it is important that both the centre and the periphery of the tumour are sampled so that variations in histological pattern can be assessed and changes in the surrounding tissue evaluated.

Mixed carcinomas displaying two or more different types occur with moderate frequency. In particular, infiltrating duct carcinoma without special features is often seen in combination with other types.

The incidence of the different types of tumour varies according to several factors, including circumstances of diagnosis (e.g. screening clinic or presentation in general population) and the country where the data are compiled.

In situ carcinoma

When a carcinoma is *in situ*, which means that the malignant cellular change is restricted to the epithelial surface, the lesion is localized and therefore is curable by resection. The absence of capillary blood vessels and lymphatics within the epithelium precludes metastasis by these routes. But it is debatable whether or not the presence of small foci of invasion can ever be definitely excluded by light microscopy, even after extensive examination of the lesion including multiple levels of multiple blocks. On electron microscopy small foci of cancer cells can be seen to protrude through defects in the basal lamina in most cases of *in situ* duct carcinoma (Ozzello, 1971).

In situ duct carcinoma

Proliferation of malignant epithelial cells within ducts can produce various histological patterns of *in situ* duct carcinoma (Figs 1.5 and 1.6), and frequently a mixed pattern is seen. Intracystic papillary carcinomas are also included under this heading. The malignant cells within the duct lumen exhibit varying degrees of cellular pleomorphism, nuclear

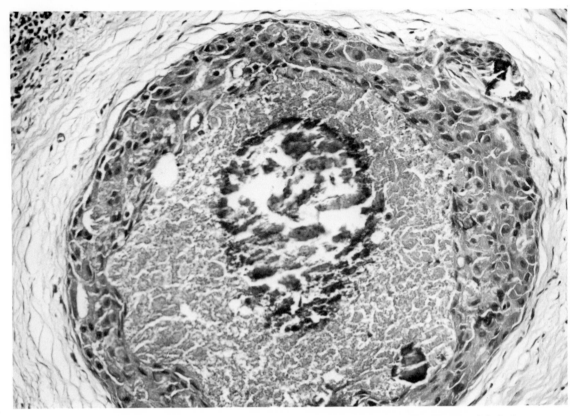

Fig. 1.5   *In situ* duct carcinoma with a comedo pattern and foci of
calcification. H and E × 240.

hyperchromasia and mitotic activity. Calcification may be present
particularly in the comedo type of *in situ* duct carcinoma when it is deposited
in the necrotic material in the centre of the mass of malignant epithelial cells
(Fig. 1.5). Spread into adjacent lobules may occur producing the so-called
'cancerization' of the lobules which must be distinguished from true *in situ*
lobular carcinoma. *In situ* duct carcinoma is frequently multifocal and this
has therapeutic implications. Patients treated by excision alone may
develop recurrent tumours. In a recent survey of the available literature
Betsill *et al.* (1978) found that at least 39% of patients subsequently
developed clinically evident carcinoma in the same breast with an average
latent period of 10 years. Very occasionally a tumour which is thought to
be purely *in situ* on microscopy is associated with metastasis in the regional
lymph nodes. This confirms the suggestion that it is not always possible to
exclude early invasion by means of light microscopy. Although *in situ* duct
carcinoma may produce a palpable mass it is frequently occult and
detection is often on the basis of mammographic calcification. It is
probably for this reason that the incidence appears to have increased

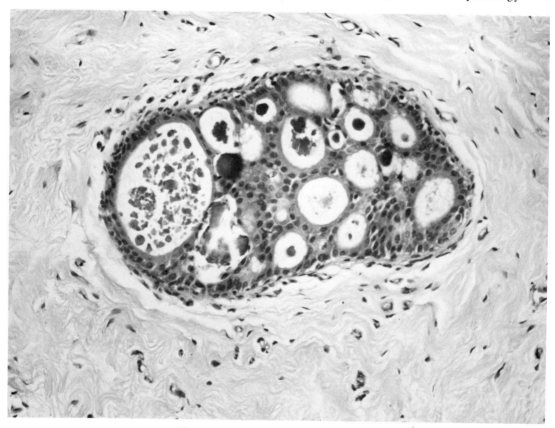

Fig. 1.6 *In situ* duct carcinoma with a cribriform pattern and foci of calcification. H and E × 240.

recently. Other modes of presentation of an impalpable *in situ* carcinoma include Paget's disease of the nipple or a blood-stained nipple discharge.

In situ lobular carcinoma

In situ lobular carcinoma was first described as a distinct form of mammary carcinoma by Foote and Stewart in 1941. The lobules are distended by fairly uniform cells which tend to lose cohesion and completely obliterate the lumina of the acini (Fig. 1.7). Spread into adjacent ducts may occur when the malignant cells infiltrate in a 'Pagetoid fashion' within the epithelial lining. *In situ* lobular carcinoma is not discernible grossly and is usually an incidental finding in biopsies performed for some other reason such as cystic disease. The overall incidence varies from 0.8–1.5% of all biopsies which are otherwise benign (Anderson, 1974; Wheeler and Enterline, 1976). Variations in incidence may be attributable partly to differences in diagnostic criteria and partly to the number of blocks prepared from biopsy specimens. There may also be

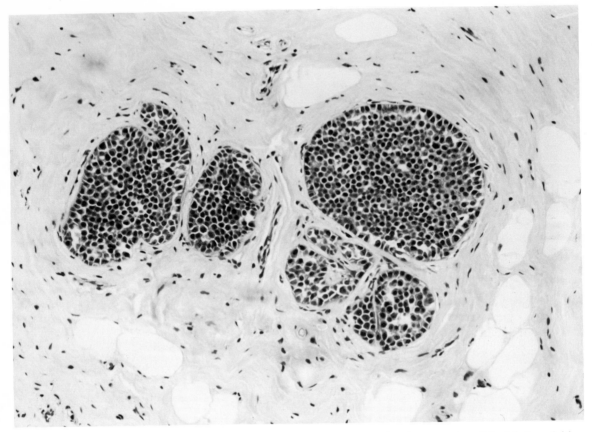

Fig. 1.7   *In situ* lobular carcinoma showing expansion of the lobular acini by rather uniform malignant cells which lack cohesion. H and E × 200.

geographical and racial differences. Occasionally *in situ* lobular carcinoma is found in tissues which have been removed because of mammographic calcification but it is rare for the calcification to be actually within the *in situ* carcinoma: it is more commonly seen in adjacent benign disease. Multifocal disease is particularly common with *in situ* lobular carcinoma and there is also a high incidence of bilaterality. Careful follow-up studies of patients treated by biopsy alone have shown that over a period of 25 years between 17 and 27% subsequently develop infiltrating carcinoma which may be of ductal or lobular type and may occur in either the ipsilateral or contralateral breast (Haagensen *et al.*, 1978; Anderson, 1977; Rosen *et al.*, 1978).

Infiltrating duct carcinoma

The majority of infiltrating carcinomas are of ductal type and almost 90% of these have no specific features. The gross appearances vary, depending

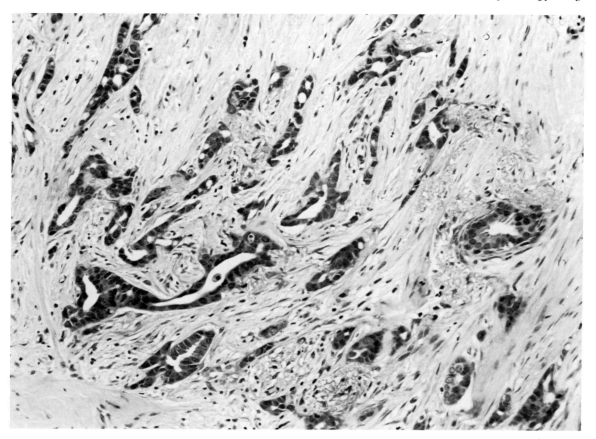

Fig. 1.8   Infiltrating duct carcinoma malignancy Grade 1. There is good tubule formation, with little nuclear pleomorphism of the malignant cells which also have a low mitotic rate. H and E × 200.

mainly on the amount and nature of the stroma, as described previously. Carcinomas with a large *in situ* component of the comedo pattern also have the typical appearance of 'comedos' exuding from the cut surface. If calcification is present within these *in situ* foci, it will be seen on a mammogram. Not infrequently, the *in situ* foci are located around the edge of the main infiltrating mass and on mammography the foci of calcification appear to be outside the main mammographic opacity.

Microscopic examination of infiltrating duct carcinoma shows malignant cells of varying size and shape, which are arranged in clusters, trabeculae or tubules (Figs 1.8 and 1.9). The amount and nature of the stroma is variable; sometimes it is densely collagenous and the centre of the tumour may be virtually acellular. In other tumours the stroma is loose and more cellular.

In situ duct carcinoma is found in association with most, but not all, infiltrating carcinomas of ductal type. In some cases no *in situ* component is seen.

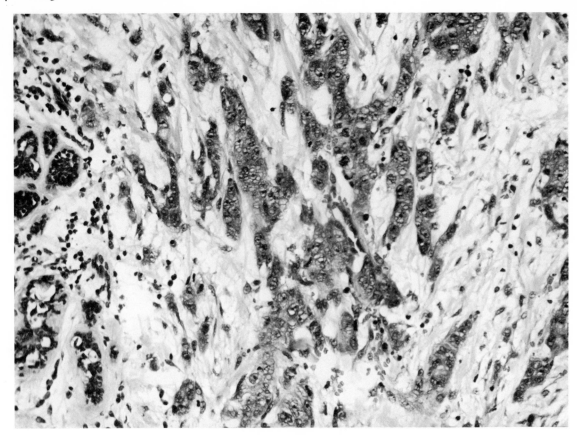

Fig. 1.9   Infiltrating duct carcinoma malignancy Grade III. There is no tubule formation. The cells exhibit marked nuclear pleomorphism and there is a high mitotic rate. H and E × 240.

Grading of infiltrating carcinoma

Some guide to the prognosis of infiltrating duct carcinomas can be obtained by grading. The system most widely used in this country is based on that described by Bloom and Richardson (1957), which takes into account three histological features: the presence or absence of tubular differentiation, the number of mitotic figures and the degree of nuclear pleomorphism of the malignant cells. The well-differentiated Grade I carcinomas show marked glandular differentiation, a low mitotic rate and little cellular pleomorphism (Fig. 1.8). Grade III carcinomas are poorly differentiated, usually with no tubular formation, marked pleomorphism and a high mitotic rate (Fig. 1.9). Grade II tumours are intermediate in differentiation. Approximately 15–20% of infiltrating duct carcinomas fall into Grade I, 20–30% are Grade III and the remaining are Grade II. The very large percentage of Grade II tumours which forms a rather hetergenous group in terms of prognosis somewhat detracts from the value of grading. Other grading systems have also been described. In the United States nuclear grading of tumours is commonly used. This can be applied to all types of mammary carcinoma. The system described by Black *et al.* (1955; 1956) originally delineated five nuclear grades, 0–4, but in more recent follow-up studies the number of grades has been reduced to 3 (Black *et al.*, 1975): poorly-differentiated nuclear Grade I tumours, moderately-differentiated nuclear Grade II and well-differentiated nuclear Grade III tumours. Thus the numerical order of this system is the reverse of the histological grading system described above and it is important to know which system of grading has been used when reading articles which refer to grading of breast carcinoma.

Special variants of duct carcinoma

Approximately 10% of infiltrating duct carcinomas comprise specific variants. Most of the tumours in this group have a more favourable prognosis than conventional duct carcinoma. As the better prognosis usually only applies if the tumour is pure and typical, strict histological criteria must be applied in diagnosis. Different types of carcinoma usually considered to be variants of infiltrating duct carcinoma include medullary carcinoma with lymphoid stroma, mucoid carcinoma, tubular carcinoma, papillary carcinoma, adenoid cystic carcinoma and carcinomas with metaplastic changes.

Medullary carcinoma. The term medullary carcinoma has been applied to any cellular tumour with a soft cut surface. In the breast it is now used to designate a particular variant of carcinoma with a heavy infiltrate of lymphocytes and plasma cells in the stroma. The term medullary carcinoma with lymphoid stroma is more accurate and precise. It usually occurs in younger women. The tumours are well defined with a rounded outline and a rather soft grey cut surface in which areas of haemorrhage and necrosis may be discernible. On both gross and mammographic examination the outline may be so smooth and rounded as to mimic a benign lesion. On histological examination the malignant cells are poorly differentiated with a high mitotic rate and are arranged in anastomizing cords and clusters with large foci of necrosis. The intervening stroma is heavily infiltrated with lymphocytes and plasma cells and lymphoid reaction centres may be present (Fig. 1.10). Even in the presence of lymph node metastases the prognosis is more favourable than would be expected from the anaplastic appearance of the malignant cells. Atypical varieties of medullary carcinoma with lymphoid stroma in which some, but not all, of the classical features are present, also have a better prognosis than the average infiltrating duct carcinoma, although the outlook is less favourable than it is with the typical form (Ridolfi *et al.*, 1977).

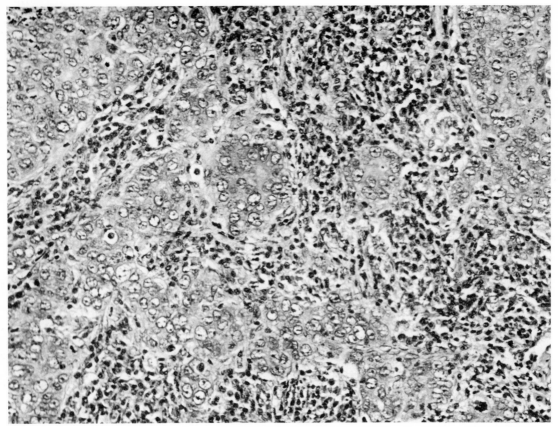

Fig. 1.10   Medullary carcinoma of breast with lymphoid stroma. Sheets of anaplastic malignant cells are surrounded by stroma which contains many lymphocytes and plasma cells. H and E × 240.

Mucoid carcinoma.   Mucoid or colloid carcinomas are characterized by large amounts of extracellular mucin, in which widely scattered groups of malignant cells appear to float (Fig. 1.11). The consistency is soft with the appearance of jelly. The outline of the tumour is usually rounded and well demarcated and the appearance may resemble a benign lesion on mammography and also sometimes on gross examination. This type of carcinoma usually occurs in older women and is associated with a better prognosis than most infiltrating duct carcinomas, but this improved outlook only applies to pure mucoid tumours.

Tubular carcinoma.   Another variant recently defined as a separate type is the tubular carcinoma. Although uncommon, tubular carcinomas are important because they are associated with a favourable prognosis. They are small and consist of uniform malignant cells arranged in tubules usually within abundant fibrous stroma. Calcification is seen fairly frequently and this, together with the irregular outline and small size, may

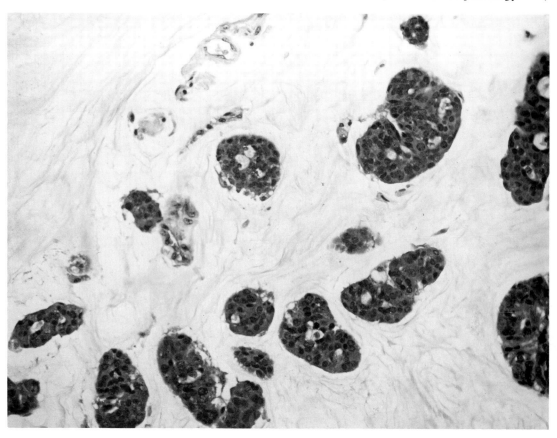

Fig. 1.11   Mucoid carcinoma of breast with islands of malignant cells surrounded by mucin. H and E × 240.

explain the relatively high detection rate of this type of carcinoma by mammography (Patchefsky *et al.*, 1977; Andersson *et al.*, 1979). Although tubular carcinomas have been regarded as a sub-type of infiltrating duct carcinoma it has been suggested recently that some may be variants of infiltrating lobular carcinoma (Eusebi *et al.*, 1979).

Infiltrating lobular carcinoma

Infiltrating lobular carcinoma probably accounts for approximately 10% of all mammary carcinomas. Microscopically the neoplastic cells vary somewhat in size from one tumour to another but are fairly uniform within the same tumour and show little pleomorphism and a low mitotic rate. Typically the cells lie singly within the stroma or are arranged in a single file ('Indian file') pattern. Sometimes the rows of cells encircle normal ducts producing the so-called 'targetoid pattern' pattern (Fig. 1.1). The amount and nature of the stroma varies as in duct carcinoma: in some it is very dense whereas in others there is little or no productive fibrosis. The term scirrhous carcinoma, used more frequently in the past, undoubtedly included some infiltrating lobular carcinomas as well as infiltrating duct carcinomas. Recently there has been increasing awareness that as well as the typical well-recognized 'targetoid', single file and single cell patterns of infiltration, other forms of infiltrating lobular carcinoma exist. This may partly account for the wide range in the reported incidence of this type of tumour, varying from 1–20% (Martinez and Azzopardi, 1979). Associated *in situ* lobular carcinoma is present in 70–80% of cases but its presence is not essential to the diagnosis. The terms small cell or round cell carcinoma usually refer to infiltrating lobular carcinoma. Most signet cell carcinomas are also considered to be variants of infiltrating lobular carcinoma, although some authorities claim they are variants of infiltrating duct carcinomas and others classify them as a separate entity (Harris *et al.*, 1978; Hull *et al.*, 1980).

Rare varieties of carcinoma

Other types of carcinoma of the breast are all relatively uncommon. Adenoid cystic carcinomas which resemble those seen in salivary glands rarely metastasize. Infiltrating carcinomas with a papillary pattern are sometimes classified separately. These tumours are well differentiated and have a relatively good prognosis. Some carcinomas have areas of metaplasia with malignant cells showing features of apocrine cells, spindle cells or squamous cells. Tumour giant cells also occur. More rarely, foci of cartilagenous or osseous metaplasia are seen. Pure squamous-cell carcinomas of the breast have also been described but are extremely rare. The prognostic significance of these metaplastic elements is uncertain (Huvos *et al.*, 1973). The type of carcinoma known as juvenile or secretory carcinoma was originally described in children but has now been recognised in adults (Norris and Taylor, 1970; Oberman, 1980). Another rare variant of mammary carcinoma is associated with the secretion of large amounts of lipid. Recently there have been several reports describing mammary carcinomas which resemble carcinoid tumours (Cubilla and Woodruff, 1977; Fisher *et al.*, 1979).

In many of these rare variants of mammary carcinoma there has been insufficient study for an accurate picture of their prognosis to be obtained.

Inflammatory carcinoma

The term inflammatory carcinoma is used more frequently by clinicians than by pathologists. Indeed, this is not really a specific pathological type of carcinoma, but a clinical picture produced by a rapidly growing tumour usually with massive involvement of the dermal lymphatics.

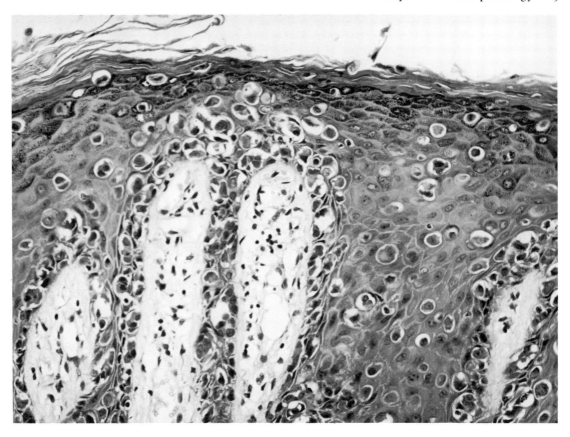

Fig. 1.12.   Paget's disease of the nipple, showing the characteristic infiltration of the epidermis with large neoplastic epithelial cells (Paget cells). H and E × 240.

Paget's disease of the nipple

Paget's disease of the nipple may occur in association with either *in situ* or infiltrating duct carcinoma. It has not been described in association with pure lobular carcinoma. Microscopically, there is permeation of the epidermis by malignant epithelial cells, scattered singly or in clumps, sometimes with tubule formation (Fig. 1.12). Mucin can frequently be demonstrated within these malignant cells. There is usually inflammation of the subjacent dermis. There is still disagreement as to whether these cells originate by direct intra-epidermal spread from an underlying carcinoma or whether they represent neoplastic change in a wide field involving both the nipple and underlying breast.

Prognostic features of infiltrating carcinoma

Various pathological features of mammary carcinoma have been correlated with prognosis. Tumour type and grade have already been mentioned. Other features, which may have prognostic significance, are related both to the appearance of the tumour itself, and to the extent of the metastatic spread. Additionally, features which are thought to represent a host-defence response to the neoplasm have been found to correlate with prognosis by some authorities.

The best known and most reliable prognostic indicator is the extent of metastatic spread. It has long been known that the presence of metastatic tumour within axillary lymph nodes indicates a significantly worse prognosis than when the nodes are not involved. Studies have also indicated that not only is the presence or absence of nodal metastases of significance, but also the number of nodes involved, the level the metastases reach in the axilla, the size of the metastases and the presence or absence of extranodal spread. Patients with less than four lymph nodes containing metastases fare considerably better than those in whom four or more nodes are involved (Fisher et al., 1968). In addition, when the involved lymph nodes are limited to the low axillary level, the prognosis is better than when nodes in the middle axillary group are involved, and when the high nodes are involved it is very likely that the tumour has already spread further (Berg, 1955; Huvos et al., 1971; Attiyeh et al., 1977). The presence of extranodal spread of metastases also has an unfavourable effect on prognosis (Fisher et al., 1976; Mambo and Gallager, 1977). Small metastases are frequently missed on routine examination, but studies in which serial sections of lymph nodes have been examined and occult metastases found have shown that the presence of these occult lesions appears to have little or no effect on prognosis (Fisher et al., 1978; Pickren, 1977).

Features of the primary tumour which have been shown to have prognostic significance, other than tumour type and grade, include the tumour size, the site within the breast, the outline of the tumour, the amount and nature of the stroma, the proportion and pattern of associated in situ carcinoma and the presence of venous invasion, lymphatic invasion or necrosis and involvement of the overlying or underlying tissues.

Recent emphasis on the importance of early detection in breast carcinoma has led to the concept of minimal breast cancer. This term was originally used to denote in situ tumours or those tumours in which the infiltrating component of the carcinoma is less than 5 mm in maximum diameter (Gallager and Martin, 1971), but some authorities also include infiltrating tumours up to 10 mm in maximum diameter (McDivitt, 1978). Such tumours are associated with a good prognosis and only rarely have axillary node metastases. With increasing use of screening techniques, particularly mammography, minimal carcinomas are now diagnosed more frequently.

The third histological component possibly related to prognosis is host resistance. This has been the subject of speculation for many years. Some authorities relate infiltration of the primary tumour by plasma cells and lymphocytes, and the presence of sinus histiocytosis in uninvolved axillary lymph nodes, with host resistance and improved survival (Hamlin, 1968; Black et al., 1955; Black et al., 1956; Silverberg et al., 1970; Black et al., 1975). Others have been unable to confirm these findings and some even claim that a marked inflammatory cell reaction to the primary tumour is associated with a poor prognosis (Champion et al., 1972; Kister et al., 1969; Fisher, 1978).

Attempts have been made to correlate many other features of the primary tumour with prognosis but unfortunately although some have initially appeared promising as independent prognostic factors, the associations have later proved to be weak or absent.

It is possible that future methods of classification of tumours and identification of prognostic indicators will relate to the demonstration of secretory metabolic products of the tumour cells, and to identifying the presence of surface antigens. Advances in immunohistochemical techniques may reveal a wide range of cellular products related to tumour type and prognosis. Development of monoclonal antibodies may make it possible to define cellular antigens associated with neoplasia and dedifferentiation.

Sarcoma

Although most malignant tumours of the breast are carcinomas derived from epithelial cells, sarcomas of mesenchymal origin also occur. Included in this group are both the malignant cystosarcoma phyllodes tumour and stromal sarcomas. Although such neoplasms are not common it is important that they should be diagnosed accurately because the treatment required is often different from that of a carcinoma. Malignant stromal tumours rarely metastasize to lymph nodes; local aggressive invasion may occur involving the chest wall and when metastasis does occur it is usually via the blood stream to lungs, liver and bones. Mammary haemangiosarcomas are another very rare but extremely malignant mesenchymal tumour. Combined carcinomas and sarcomas can occur in the breast but are very uncommon.

Lymphoma and leukaemia

The breast may be involved by malignant lymphoma as part of a disseminated disease, but a few cases of primary lymphoma limited to the breast have been described. Leukaemic involvement of the breast can also occur.

Metastatic tumours

Secondary tumours of the breast other than lymphoma are unusual but any malignant tumour can metastasize to the breast; the most common are carcinoma of the lung, malignant melanoma and ovarian carcinoma. On gross examination metastatic tumours are usually rounded and sharply demarcated from the surrounding tissue. Their appearance on mammography is deceptive, resembling a benign lesion (McIntosh *et al.*, 1976). If the tumour is well differentiated and resembles the primary source there is no difficulty in histological diagnosis. But anaplastic secondary tumours may be difficult to distinguish from undifferentiated primary breast carcinoma, particularly on frozen section. Close collaboration between clinician and pathologist is crucial, and when another primary tumour is known to exist the pathologist must be told.

Metastatic carcinoma from the contralateral breast may also be difficult to differentiate from a second primary. A confident diagnosis of a second primary carcinoma can only be made if there is contiguous *in situ* change, the second tumour is of a different type or if it is better differentiated than the first carcinoma.

CLASSIFICATION OF BENIGN BREAST DISEASE

The classification of benign diseases of the breast is as controversial as that for malignant tumours. Again most of the disagreement is over terminology. For the purposes of this chapter there is no need for a comprehensive account of benign breast disease but it is worth considering some of the more common conditions particularly those which may be mistaken on clinical, gross or microscopic examination for malignant lesions.

Cystic hyperplasia

Many benign breast lesions form distinct entities and are therefore easily classified, for example, fibroadenoma and duct ectasia. However, other conditions which are largely characterized by a spectrum of proliferative and involutionary changes within the glandular tissue of the breast are usually lumped together under a variety of headings: benign mammary dysplasia, fibroadenosis or fibrocystic disease being the most common. All the used terms have been criticized. Some people object to the use of the word dysplasia because it has a connotation of premalignancy when applied to certain other structures, such as cervix uteri. Fibrocystic disease and fibroadenosis tend to suggest specific changes which may or may not be present in all examples. The term cystic hyperplasia has been suggested by Azzopardi (1979a) because this indicates both the most common and probably the most important changes found. Studies of the relationship between benign breast disease and malignancy have demonstrated a slight but definite increase in risk associated with cystic hyperplasia (Azzopardi, 1979b). Judging from recent work this risk appears to be associated only with those lesions which show epithelial hyperplasia (Page *et al.*, 1978; Wellings *et al.*, 1975; Hutchinson *et al.*, 1980).

Epithelial hyperplasia occurs both in ducts and lobules. Although frequently associated with the presence of cysts it can occur in isolation. The proliferation of epithelial cells may result in partial or total obliteration of the lumen and sometimes numerous luminal spaces are present within otherwise solid sheets of proliferating cells. This appearance is sometimes called papillomatosis. Differential diagnosis from *in situ* duct carcinoma is sometimes very difficult. Similarly epithelial hyperplasia in lobules can produce difficulties in differentiation from *in situ* lobular carcinoma.

Cysts which may be single or multiple can produce a very firm mass often considered clinically to be a carcinoma. On gross examination the true nature of the lesion is usually evident but microscopically a brisk surrounding fibroblastic reaction and chronic inflammatory cell infiltration, which may result from leakage of cyst contents, can be confused with infiltrating malignant cells, particularly on frozen section.

Sclerosing adenosis

The term adenosis has been used to describe both an increase in the number of tubular structures, probably derived from lobules, and alterations in the architecture of these lobular structures. The most important and commonest variety, sclerosing adenosis, is characterized by a localized proliferation of epithelial and myoepithelial cells as well as stroma. Excessive fibrosis with hyalinization and sometimes associated elastosis in such lesions can result in a stellate appearance which may be mistaken on both gross and mammographic examination for a carcinoma. The not infrequent presence of calcification adds to the resemblance. Microscopically also differentiation from carcinoma can be difficult because of disorganization of breast architecture. A variety of terms have been used to describe these sclerotic scar-like lesions including sclerosing papillary proliferation, sclerosing adenosis with pseudo-infiltration and infiltrating epitheliosis (Azzopardi, 1979c).

Duct ectasia

Duct ectasia (periductal mastitis, plasma cell mastitis, comedo mastitis or obliterative mastitis) is characterized by progressive dilatation of the mammary duct system, usually commencing beneath the nipple. In its earliest stages the dilated ducts are surrounded by chronic inflammatory cells including a high proportion of plasma cells; in the later stages the duct wall is fibrotic and the epithelium may be entirely missing. Tenacious green material is present within the lumen of the ducts and calcification may occur either within the lumen or in a ring-like fashion within the walls. The appearance of the calcification on mammography is usually diagnostic but can sometimes closely mimic *in situ* duct carcinoma. Duct ectasia can produce nipple retraction and is maybe associated with a blood-stained nipple discharge.

Duct papilloma

Another benign lesion which often presents with a blood-stained nipple discharge is a benign duct papilloma. This may arise anywhere within the ductal system but is most commonly found immediately beneath the nipple and consists of papillary structures with well-developed fibrous cores covered by epithelium and myoepithelium. Although there may be mild hyperplasia of the epithelium the cells are regularly arranged and the myoepithelium is easily identifiable. Areas of apocrine metaplasia are not infrequently present. Most benign duct papillomas present no diagnostic problems but occasionally differentiation from an intracystic papillary carcinoma is difficult.

Fibroadenoma

Fibroadenomas are discrete benign lesions formed by proliferation of both connective tissue and epithelial elements. The epithelial moiety can exhibit a variety of changes: apocrine metaplasia, sclerosing adenosis, hyperplasia and very rarely carcinoma, usually of lobular type. The connective tissue component may be densely collagenous or loose and extremely myxoid; it may feature replacement by adipose tissue and foci of calcification or even ossification. Malignant change within the stromal element can also occur but again is rare and usually only seen in the special variety of fibroadenoma, the so-called cystosarcoma phyllodes tumour.

Adenoma

Pure adenomas of the breast are uncommon, well-defined benign lesions, composed of epithelial elements with inconspicuous stroma.

Other benign neoplasms

Other benign soft tissue tumours of the breast, apart from the lipoma are extremely rare. The latter usually present no diagnostic problems. A lesion which has been recognized recently, because of its distinctive appearance on mammography, is the so-called mammary hamartoma (Hessler et al., 1978; Linell et al., 1979). This lesion appears as a well-circumscribed homogeneous mass on mammography and is usually diagnosed clinically as a fibroadenoma but is softer on gross examination. Microscopically the lesion appears as a well-demarcated mass of mammary ducts and lobules within varying amounts of fibrous stroma and adipose tissue. The changes of cystic hyperplasia may be present. The lesion is not a true hamartoma in the sense of a tumour-like malformation.

Fat necrosis

Fat necrosis is another benign condition which may be confused with carcinoma both on clinical and mammographic examination. There is usually a history of trauma but sometimes no such history can be elicited, particularly in women with large, fatty breasts. There may be skin tethering and dimpling and a range of mammographic appearances have been described including changes which may mimic a carcinoma (Bassett *et al.*, 1978). The macroscopic appearances are usually characteristic with the opaque, bright yellow necrotic fat contrasting with the paler, translucent normal adipose tissue. On histological examination the necrotic fat is surrounded by foamy macrophages, reactive fibroblasts and often foreign body giant cells.

CONCLUSION

Problems of histological interpretation can arise in all fields of pathology but the breast presents the pathologist with some of the most difficult differential diagnoses. Close co-operation between pathologist and clinician is particularly important in this field. It is essential that the pathologist is fully aware of the clinical situation and the reason for the biopsy. The surgeon should be aware of the limitations of pathological examination and supply the pathologist with as much relevant information as possible. An effort should always be made to ensure that the pathological findings correlate with and explain the clinical and mammographic features. If there is any discrepancy, consideration must be given to the possibility that the biopsy sample has not been adequately examined or that the extent of the surgery has been insufficient to include the lesional tissue within the biopsy specimen.

2

CLINICAL FEATURES OF BREAST DISEASE

J.A. McKinna

CLINICAL ASSESSMENT

Clinical assessment of the breast is based, as in all other organ or body systems, on the history and careful physical examination. This is carried out in the knowledge that all women presenting with breast symptoms are anxious that they may have cancer.

Historical features

The most important historical features to be considered are present symptomatology, age and menstrual status, hormone manipulation (and other medication), previous breast disease and family history.

Present symptomatology

It is best to allow a woman to describe in her own words the symptoms which are causing her concern, and of the way in which she made the discovery.

The presence of mass. The discovery of a mass in the breast is very frightening for the patient, and, women will vary in their reactions to it. The patient's attitude is dependent upon her personality and on the imagined consequences of treatment, which leads some to postpone the necessary medical examination which may make the diagnosis and solve the problem. Others seek help immediately from their family doctor who has the responsibility of primary examination and diagnosis and of making a decision about specialist referral. More breast lumps are benign than malignant, and many are not serious. However, many general practitioners will feel that reassurance comes best from a specialist who has the support of additional diagnostic services.

Multiplicity of masses or generalized lumpiness. In women 25–30% have diffusely lumpy breasts. This change may be confined to one quadrant, usually the upper outer, or it may involve larger amounts of one or both breasts. The consistency is related to the amount of fibrous tissue stroma and to the thickness of the overlying fat. If such breasts are biopsied, these patients are found to have varying degrees of benign mammary dysplasia. Women who practise regular self-examination will be aware of this nodularity and they are the best observers to appreciate or detect an alteration – such as the appearance of a new, dominant lump. Many women with such changes find them distasteful and frightening and some ignore them while others seek regular medical reassurance (Gray, 1981).

Pain and tenderness.   Pain and tenderness are common breast symptoms and when localized, may be associated with a mass. Acute pain is suggestive of a sudden change, such as the rapid distension of a simple cyst, and on occasions this may be quite severe. However, severe pain in the breast is usually related to inflammatory pathology and will be greatest when it occurs near the surface with involvement of the skin and subcutaneous fat and its generous nerve supply.

Pain is not a frequent symptom in cancer, although about 20% of women with cancer will experience some discomfort in the breast which can be related to the tumour. The commonest painful symptom of a tumour is usually described as a pricking sensation, and this may be quite significant if it is localized to the area of a palpable lump. It is much more common for tumours to progress slowly within the breast without causing any pain at all. Under these circumstances, pain, or the lack of it, is related to the rate of change of the tissues and some tumours can grow to quite large proportions without causing any pain or abnormal sensation.

Cyclical changes.   Cyclical symptoms in the breast related to menstruation are very common and might be regarded as physiological. Many women experience swelling of the breast in the premenstrual days. This is associated with increased mammary bloodflow in response to changes in hormone levels and normally lasts only a day or two. Under the pathological circumstances of the premenstrual syndrome in which there is a deficiency of progesterone in the second half of the cycle, the symptoms may persist for two weeks. This situation may be relieved by the administration of a progesterone, by Vitamin B_6 (Pyridoxine) in large dosage or by a diuretic. It is an important part of clinical assessment to know that such changes occur and to relate the findings at examination to the time in the patient's menstrual cycle.

Change in breast size.   Some patients with proliferative breast lesions (either benign or malignant) experience an increase in size of the breast rather than the detection of a single lump or even of nodularity. This is not a common symptom but it is one which causes concern, particularly if it is unilateral. Symmetrical decrease in size due to atrophy and ptosis is commonly seen after pregnancy and lactation and after the menopause.

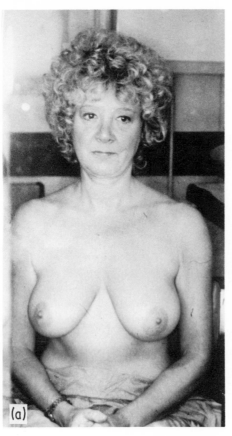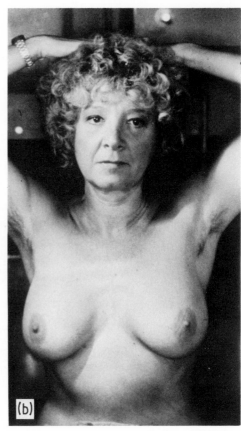

Fig. 2.1   The woman inspects her breasts in the mirror with arms at her side (a) and raised (b).

Change in shape.   The doctor examining a patient who has observed a change in the shape of the breast must remember that she is making the observation face on in the mirror as well as from above (Figs 2.1 and 2.2). The most important change in shape which always requires full evaluation is the appearance of a dimple in the skin, which may be caused by the retraction of a fibrous strand from an underlying tumour.

Nipple abnormality.   The common nipple changes which require examination and investigation are retraction, ulceration or discharge.

A nipple which withdraws, but which can be manipulated to protrude normally, is described as being retractile, and, one which flattens or disappears without any re-emergence is retracted. It is important to discover whether this retraction is due to attachment to underlying disease, which is most often carcinoma but may be inflammatory and associated with duct ectasia or plasma cell mastitis.

Ulceration of the nipple is not a common condition and may be simply eczematous or the first sign of Paget's disease.

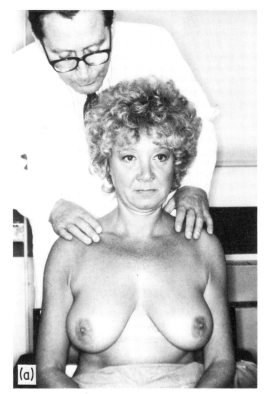 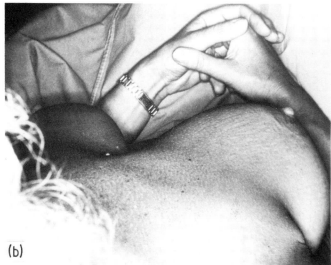

Fig. 2.2   The doctor should inspect the breasts from above the patient's shoulder (a) seeing the breasts from above (b).

Discharge from the nipple may be associated with ulceration but usually comes from one of the major ducts. It is important to identify the colour of the discharge and its relation to menstrual changes and to previous lactation. Bloodstained discharge from a single duct is often the only sign of a simple duct papilloma. Brown or green discharge from a number of ducts is usually due to benign fibrocystic disease involving and communicating with the major duct system.

Axillary pain or swelling.   A major part of the regional lymphatic drainage of the breast is situated in the axilla where lymph node enlargement due to tumour or associated with an inflammatory breast condition is a common finding. Discomfort in the axilla may be cyclical or associated with a wide variety of breast problems.

Age of menstrual status

The age of the patient is helpful in establishing priorities in the differential diagnosis. In affluent Western society, the age-specific incidence of breast cancer rises with increasing years. Breast cancer is an uncommon disease in women under the age of 30, but, of course, cancer should not be excluded as a possible diagnosis merely on grounds of the patient's youthfulness. Indeed, one of the distressing features about carcinoma of the breast in young women is the delay in diagnosis which can be caused by inappropriate reassurance.

It is important to relate the cyclical variations in breast activity to the specific symptoms and to understand the background which they contribute to the diseased breast. Such changes continue up to the time of the menopause. Women who have had hysterectomy with ovarian conservation will of course continue to have cyclical ovarian activity and associated breast changes may occur.

Hormone manipulation

During and after the menopause, cyclical breast changes usually regress but stimulation of breast tissue and breast activity is now seen in those taking hormone replacement therapy for distressing menopausal symptoms. If the treatment is of a cyclical type, then the corresponding breast changes may well be cyclical. Some women who had mastalgia during their reproductive life will report a recurrence of breast pain following the start of such therapy. There is no proven association between the incidence of breast cancer and hormone replacement therapy. There has always been a considerable anxiety about the prolonged use of unopposed oestrogen as a possible aetiological factor of breast carcinoma in postmenopausal women. There is so far no convincing data to show that this actually occurs, but there is no doubt that oestrogens will stimulate some breast tumours that already exist. Current evidence suggests that the uterine endothelium should be stimulated with physiological doses of oestrogen and progesterone in a cyclical way rather than by unopposed oestrogen since there is a real risk of inducing carcinoma of the corpus uteri in these circumstances. It will be interesting to follow the incidence of breast cancer in women taking hormone replacement therapy in this more physiological way.

The contraceptive pill, of course, is the most frequent exogenous source of cyclical female hormones. There is no evidence (Vessey *et al.* 1981) that the prolonged use of the contraceptive pill is related to an increased incidence of breast cancer. Epidemiologists will point out that the contraceptive pill has not been in existence for the 25–30 years which may be necessary to see an increase in breast cancer due to its use. As a general rule, the pill diminishes breast discomfort and nodularity, but may be associated with an increase in breast size. Absence of any change in breast size or cyclical discomfort is also quite common. Rarely, the use of the contraceptive pill causes the breasts to be more active and lumpier than they had been prior to its administration. In the early years of experience with oral contraceptives, such women were often described as having 'pill breasts' and the incidence of such nodular changes seems to have fallen along with the reduction in oestrogen dosage in most forms of contraceptive pill.

It is important to enquire about other hormones which the patient may be taking for gynaecological reasons. It is quite common to treat women with premenstrual symptoms with a progesterone. This may reduce mastalgia and nodularity in the pre-menstrual breast and it is important to know about this. Bromocryptine is an inhibitor of prolactin synthesis and it may reduce breast activity, particularly in those patients where that activity is associated with hyperprolactinaemia. Danazole inhibits the pituitary production of follicular stimulating hormone and luteinizing hormone and this inhibition may have a secondary effect in reducing the glandular activity of the breast.

Previous breast disease

A history of benign breast disease, which may or may not have required surgery, is important in establishing the background for new breast pathology, and in making the differential diagnosis more comprehensive. Women who have had a benign biopsy which showed simple fibroadenosis may present with a new swelling in the breast which has the clinical features of benign disease. The earlier benign biopsy increases the likelihood of a similar diagnosis on this occasion. However, if the benign biopsy showed significant epithelial hyperplasia or intraduct papillomatosis, the clinician is alerted to the increased risk of malignancy since these conditions are thought to be premalignant. Many attempts have been made to quantify the risk of developing breast cancer in relation to previous benign disease and the difficulties are at least twofold. The first is that benign breast disease is not a single condition and the important premalignant feature seems to be epithelial hyperplasia, which is not present in every case. Secondly, it is quite difficult to establish a prospective study in which the incidence of breast cancer in women with benign disease is compared with a control population who have no evidence of benign disease but in whom other predisposing factors are identical. Women with symptoms of benign disease are examined more frequently and tend to have more frequent surgical biopsies and this leads to a higher cancer detection rate.

Family history

There are many reports in the literature demonstrating the increased incidence of breast cancer in female relatives of women who have had the disease. This is higher than would be expected in the general population by a factor of two. When the lifetime risk in our society of the development of breast cancer is approximately 1 in 15, that risk will be doubled to approximately 1 in 8 in women with a family history of breast cancer on the maternal side. Anderson (1971 and 1974) has shown that this risk is increased for daughters of women who developed the disease before the menopause by 4.6 times, and for sisters of women with breast cancer appearing before the menopause by 2.7 times.

Nulliparous women have a 1.5 times increased risk of developing breast cancer compared with the general population and this will enhance the familial risk. The appearance of breast carcinoma in such women is described as occurring up to 10 years earlier than it did in the affected relative. Unmarried women whose mothers and sisters have had breast cancer are at greatest risk of developing the disease and wherever possible should be included in screening programmes so that the disease can be detected whilst it is still curable. We have found in our studies in the Early Diagnostic Unit of The Royal Marsden Hospital that there is an increased frequency of bilateral disease, which may be synchronous or metachronous, in women with a family history and this confirms the findings of others including those in Anderson's large series.

The presence of such a family history should alert the clinician to an increased degree of anxiety on the part of the patient and, possibly, to a greater need for decisions about biopsy and for firm reassurance if biopsy is not indicated.

Physical examination

Inspection

The woman should sit, unclothed to the waist, in a good light facing the examiner. He should inspect the shape, size and symmetry of both breasts and nipples. She should then gradually raise her arms sideways above her head, any differences between the sides are noted. As she brings her arms down, she should be asked to place them on the hips with resulting pectoral contraction.

Haagensen has drawn attention to the usefulness of inspecting the patient leaning forward towards the examiner, allowing the breasts to fall away from the chest wall (Fig. 2.3). This may demonstrate an otherwise hidden asymmetry and it certainly has the advantage of encouraging the doctor to look at the breasts from above, just as the patient does herself.

Important points to look for in inspection of the breasts are symmetry, skin changes, and nipple changes.

Symmetry. It is important to examine the shape and size of the breasts in relation to each other. It is not uncommon for there to be a slight difference in size between the left and right breast, but it is important to know if this is of recent origin. Similarly, one could be interested in the cyclical variations which the patient has noted.

The presence of a mass in the breast may be visible to the patient and to the examiner. In order to be visible, the lump has to be near the skin or of a considerable size in relation to the breast in which it lies (Fig. 2.4). Lumps

Fig. 2.3   When the patient leans
forward the breasts can be examined
from the chest wall.

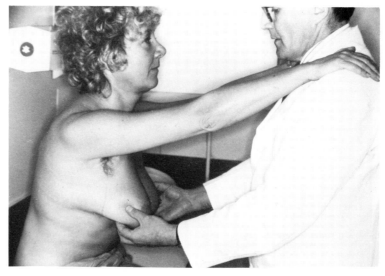

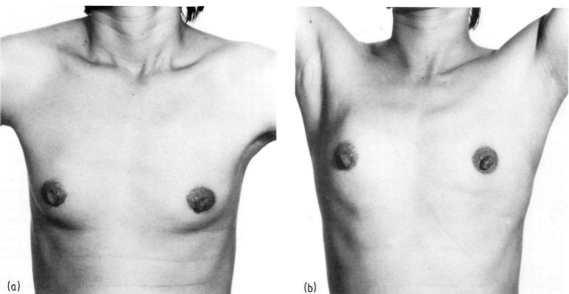

(a)

(b)

Fig. 2.4   The mass in the upper half of the right breast of this 31-year-old
Filipino (a) is much more easily seen when she raises her arms (b).

are sometimes visible in the axilla. The commonest cause of **axillary
asymmetry** and of a lump in the axilla is the presence of excess **fat in or**
above the axillary tail, in essence this produces an axillary lipoma **which is**
not localized and which, on histological examination, will contain **strands**
of breast tissue.

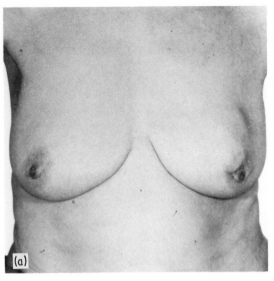
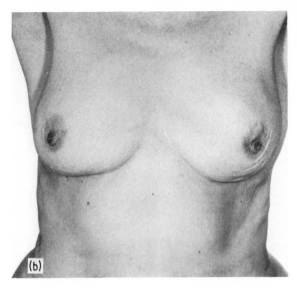

Fig. 2.5   This 67-year-old woman has a visible and palpable mass above the left nipple (a) and skin furrows appear below the nipple when she raises her arm (b).

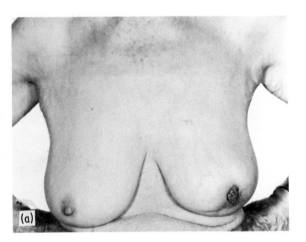
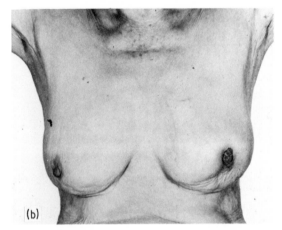

Fig. 2.6   The central tumour in this woman's left breast has produced central fixation of the nipple in a contracted areola ('Circumvallate' nipple) (a); the atrophic skin furrows below both nipples are well seen when she raises her arms but, the skin tethering of the tumour deforms them on the left (b).

Skin changes.   Changes in the skin such as a dimple or a groove often indicates underlying pathology. If single and asymmetrical, this is usually associated with an underlying carcinoma (Fig. 2.5), but, it must be remembered that creases in the skin of the atrophic postmenopausal breast

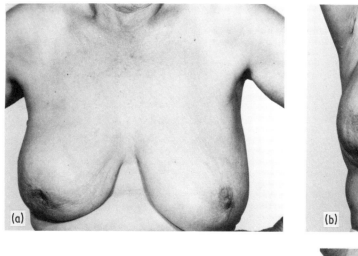

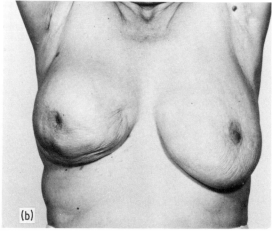

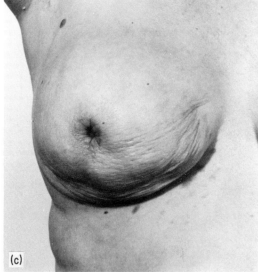

Fig. 2.7   The large tumour in this woman's right breast has caused asymmetry (a), skin tethering in several areas (b) and retraction of the nipple with oedema of the skin below it (peau d'orange) (c). There is a linear crease in the right axilla (b) where skin is tethered to malignant nodes (showing extranodal extension).

are often seen (Fig. 2.6) and they may also be seen in women who have had a sudden recent loss in weight for whatever reason. Oedema of the skin which may indicate a failure of dermal lymphatic drainage is characterized by a peau d'orange appearance in its grossest form (Fig. 2.7). Lesser degrees of oedema may not be visible, but may be palpable as an increase in thickness of the skin with a loss of elasticity compared with the surrounding normal skin. There may be vascular changes in the skin with erythema and with prominence of subcutaneous veins. These skin changes may be additional to a visible mass or may draw attention to a palpable abnormality. Advanced tumours infiltrate the skin by direct extension (Fig. 2.8).

Prominent veins are often visible to the examining clinician but may be

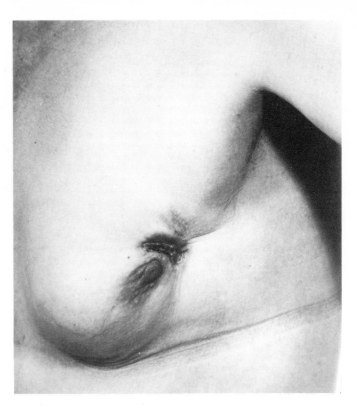

Fig. 2.8   Nipple retraction towards a carcinoma which has directly infiltrated the skin.

best demonstrated by thermography or infra-red photography. Both of these examinations may also show increased circulatory changes which are not necessarily associated with any visible erythema. A well-recognized venous condition is Mondor's disease, in which one of the subcutaneous veins of the breast undergoes thrombosis. It used to be taught that this was an infallible sign of malignancy but it does also occur in the absence of carcinoma. In the latter case, the condition resolves spontaneously without treatment over a period of a few weeks and during that time, the linear groove in the skin overlying the thrombosed vein is a very dramatic physical sign.

Nipple changes.   The visible changes in the nipple are those which have already been referred to in the historical section, namely, retraction, ulceration or discharge. The nipples may be congenitally retracted on one side or both. The most common causes of acquired nipple retraction are underlying carcinoma (Figs 2.6 and 2.7) and duct ectasia. Retraction may be caused by a tumour which is not immediately under the nipple but in which there is periductal spread and fibrosis. The pathogenesis of retraction of nipple or skin is almost always related to the contraction of fibrous tissue. However, central retraction of the nipple is sometimes associated with oedema of the nipple–areolar complex and this may result in 'circumvallate' appearance (Fig. 2.6).

The normal nipple may be associated with a very minor degree of crusting and epithelial replacement. Sometimes this is excessive and the nipple is heavily crusted. This is not a sign of any underlying pathology, particularly, if it is symmetrical, but, recent crusting of one side may be one of the first signs of Paget's disease of the nipple. Paget's disease may resemble eczema with epithelial thickening and erythema. Most commonly it is associated with some degree of ulceration. Typically, this will start on the central ductal part of the nipple and very gradually progress outward along the nipple surface and on to the areola (Fig. 2.9). This is only very slowly progressive and may eventually involve the periareolar skin, usually after several years (Fig. 2.10).

Palpation

Gentle palpation of each breast in a systematic manner will follow inspection. This can be begun whilst the patient is sitting and is a convenient time to ask her what position she was in when the lump was first noticed, many are found in the upright position in the bath or shower. Palpation of the axilla is best effected in the upright position but in general, palpation of the breast should be carried out with the patient supine.

The important parts of the examination comprise palpation of the breast, the skin and the regional lymph nodes.

The breast. When the patient lies in the supine position with her arms resting on the pillow above her head, the breasts may be examined more systematically and symmetrically. If she has a dominant lump, the examination can be started at this site and then the other segments of the breast should be felt using the 'flat of the hand', that is the palmar aspects of the distal and middle phalanges (Fig. 2.11). This is important in the assessment of the general configuration of the breast tissue, and the pressure of the examining hand will determine the depth of perception; this will also be dependent on the size and consistency of the breast and the relative proportions of fat and glandular tissue. It is a matter of personal preference whether one examines a dominant lump first in detail or whether one returns to it after a careful assessment of the remaining tissue of both breasts. The latter approach will give a better general impression of the breast type which may be related to the palpable pathology and later related to mammography.

If a lump is found in the breast, it is important to make note of the classical physical signs of a lump, namely the site, size, shape and surface, consistency, mobility and attachments and the regional lymph node drainage. Benign breast lumps such as fibroadenomata and simple cysts are often smooth and mobile. The mobility of a breast lump depends on the density of the tissue in which it is situated and the attachments between it and that tissue. A classical fibroadenoma is a smooth ovoid mass, often approximately 1 cm in diameter which is freely mobile within

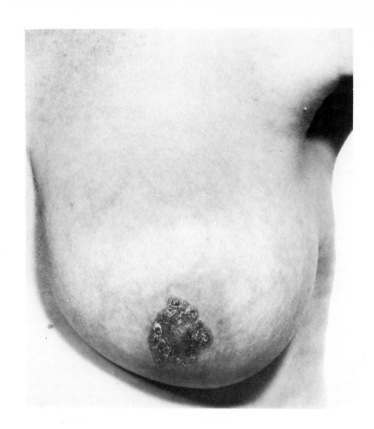

Fig. 2.9 Paget's disease of the left
nipple.

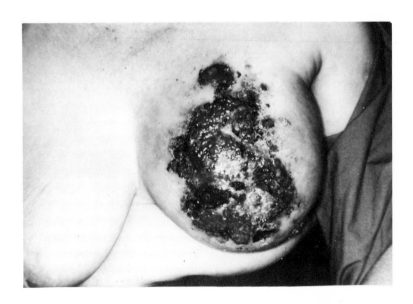

Fig. 2.10 Extensive Paget's disease
involving the skin of the breast.

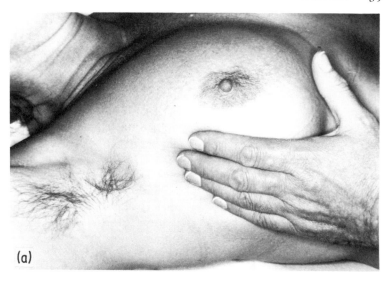

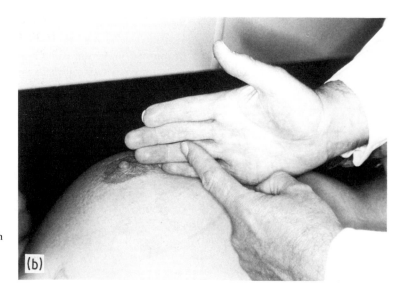

Fig. 2.11   The breast is examined with the flat of the hand (a) using the palmar surface of distal and middle phalanges (b).

the breast and commonly described as a 'breast mouse'. However, such a swelling may be present within the substance of the breast tissue and not freely mobile. This does not indicate any malignancy but merely that it is restrained by stromal attachment.

Malignant tumours of the breast are commonly hard and irregular, but there are exceptions to those general characteristics. The consistency of a tumour is a function of the amount of fibrous tissue within it, the more fibrous tissue the harder the tumour. The hardness or firmness of the tumour is also a function of the difference between it and the surrounding fat or breast tissue. This distinction between the firmness of the pathological lesion and the surrounding breast tissue is particularly important in the commonest lumpy condition of the breast, that is, fibroadenosis. This benign process is a mixture of varying proportions of fibrosis and adenosis with microcyst formation and is sometimes associated with major cysts. It is one of the common ways in which the breast ages and the condition may be generalized throughout both breasts or it may be localized to one segment, or even a small area of one breast. The firmness is a function of the proportion of fibrous tissue and this may be different in various areas of the pathological process. This is similar to the radiological evidence of dysplasia which may also show single or multiple areas of discrete involvement or a diffuse change. Benign mammary dysplasia is a 'portmanteau' term to incorporate all forms of fibroadenosis, benign proliferative conditions and benign tumours of the breast (Scarff and Torloni, 1968).

It is important that after gently and carefully palpating each quadrant of the breast to examine the central ductal tissue under the nipple. If there is any discharge it will be expressed at this time and it will be appreciated whether it comes from one duct or many, and the colour and nature of the discharge can be fully investigated.

Emphasis on gentle palpation is important since many women have tender breasts, this is especially true of younger women who are examined in the premenstrual phase of their cycle. A localized area of tenderness should be examined with great care. In general, pain and tenderness are symptoms of benign disease such as active fibroadenosis or inflammatory conditions rather than of malignant disease. However, the symptom and

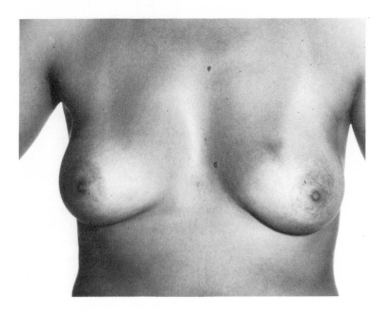

Fig. 2.12   There is discoloration of the skin in the upper inner quadrant of the left breast overlying a firm irregular area of fat necrosis.

the sign tend to be associated and if a malignant tumour is painful, it is usually tender as well.

The skin. If there are changes in the skin, one will be determining by palpation if skin thickening or oedema are present since minimal degrees of oedema are more easily felt than seen (Fig. 2.12). Similarly, infiltration of the skin by tumour is a visible sign but may be detected earlier by palpation. Dimples which are related to underlying adherent tumours can be demonstrated more easily when the tumour is manipulated between the fingers and the skin dimple made more or less obvious. The presence of an inflammatory condition which may be suspected because of increased vascularity will be related also to an increase in skin temperature which is best appreciated using the extensor surfaces of the fingers.

CLINICAL FEATURES OF BENIGN AND MALIGNANT CONDITIONS

Benign mammary dysplasia

Cysts. The physical signs of a cyst in the breast are usually those of a rounded mass with a smooth surface, this is especially true if its surface is covered by only a thin layer of fat and not by dense, nodular breast tissue. The size of a cyst can vary from a few millimetes in diameter to several centimetres and its volume may vary from less than 1 ml to 50 ml or more. The consistency is a function of the tension of fluid within the cyst and its mobility is a function of the attachments of the cyst wall to the surrounding breast tissue. A solitary thin-walled cyst within a fatty breast will be very mobile, whilst, a cyst lying within firm fibrous breast tissue with only its superficial aspect accessible, may not be palpable at all. The rate of development is extremely variable, some cysts will become apparent overnight and others may remain unchanged within the breast for several months or years. Simple cysts may be single or multiple.

The diagnosis is confirmed by fine needle aspiration. The fluid from a benign cyst may be clear or cloudy, and yellow, brown or pale green. Some cysts contain thick pseudopurulent secretions which are the consistency of condensed milk. A blood-stained aspirate may be due to a papillary tumour arising in the lining of the cyst or due to invasion by an adjacent carcinoma. In general, cytology of colourless or yellow fluid aspirated from a cyst is unrewarding.

Fibroadenosis with multiple microcyst formation. This is the commonest form of nodular change in the breasts and it may be localized to one segment of one breast, or a diffuse change throughout both breasts. The firmness to palpation is a function of the amount of fibrous tissue within it. Clinical examination will not yield any information about the nature of the adenosis, nor about any epithelial hyperplasia, which will only be revealed by biopsy.

Fibrous mastopathy (sclerosing mastopathy or fibrosclerosis).   This is the firmest form of benign mammary dysplasia and may produce quite a hard lump which can be indistinguishable from a carcinoma on clinical examination. Fine needle aspiration demonstrates that such tissue resists the introduction of a needle even more than most carcinomas: the fibrous breast tissue grips the needle, which may even bend. This physical sign is almost always associated with benign fibrous breast disease.

Sclerosing adenosis.   This is a histological diagnosis which mimics carcinoma clinically, radiologically, cytologically and pathologically. The clinical features are those of a localized firm mass which may be slightly irregular. This can be related to a spiculated disturbance of architecture seen on mammography, and also seen on naked eye section of the lump at surgical biopsy. The histological features of this condition may also prove difficult to distinguish from well differentiated intraduct carcinoma with a fibrous stroma.

Duct ectasia.   Dilatation of major or minor ducts within the breast lead to retention of secretions within them. This secretion may leak from the ducts and produce an inflammatory reaction. This, in turn, produces a lump which may be similar to a carcinoma on palpation. It commonly occurs in the tissue immediately under the nipple–areolar complex and may be associated with nipple retraction. There may be radiological or cytological evidence which allows duct ectasia to be distinguished from carcinoma, but open biopsy will often be the only reliable method of making the distinction.

Acute mastitis and abscess.   Acute inflammatory conditions of the breast caused by bacterial infection occur most commonly but not exclusively in the lactating or postpartum breast. They are associated with the symptoms and signs of acute inflammation, namely pain and tenderness, a local increase in temperature of the affected segment of the breast and erythema of the skin overlying it. The infection may be a diffuse parenchymatous process or it may consist of pus within an infected galactocele. The diagnosis will be confirmed by fine needle aspiration or by incision and drainage.

Galactocele.   This is a condition describing cyst formation within a lactating breast. The cyst is full of milk and although it can be aspirated, this may have to be done on several occasions in order to allow the walls of the cyst to adhere one to the other, thus obliterating the space.

Fat necrosis.   This occurs in response to trauma and the commonest demonstration of it is seen in the breast following surgical biopsy. However, 'spontaneous' fat necrosis does occur and it causes the detection of a firm, irregular mass in the breast which mimics a carcinoma.

Gynaecomastia.   This is a benign, proliferative epithelial disorder of the male breast which will produce an irregular lump, often tender and painful, under the nipple. It is often associated with a hormonal disturbance such as treatment with oestrogens for the management of carcinoma of the prostate, liver dysfunction or some other disturbance of oestrogen catabolism.

Benign tumours of the breast

Adenoma of the breast.   A true adenoma, as distinct from a fibroadenoma, is an uncommon entity and histologically, the epithelial element resembles that of a pericanalicular fibroadenoma, but there is a minimal stroma within the tumour which is usually well encapsulated. Clinically, it is indistinguishable from the more common fibroadenoma.

Adenoma of the nipple.   This condition resembles a sweat gland adenoma, and is a papillary lesion on the nipple. It may be indistinguishable from Paget's disease and the condition, although papillary, does not resemble a duct papilloma.

Duct papilloma.   This is a solitary papillary benign lesion growing in one of the main ducts close to the nipple. It usually presents with a serous or blood-stained discharge from a single duct on the nipple surface. The diagnosis may be confirmed by galactography prior to excision of the affected duct and segment of breast tissue.

Fibroadenoma.   This is a benign mobile tumour commonly encapsulated and containing hyperplastic epithelium and hyperplastic fibrous tissue. There are two variants histologically, (a) pericanalicular fibroadenoma and (b) intracanalicular fibroadenoma. The former is usually hard and the latter soft. Each of these tumours is commonly mobile and may be so freely mobile, in a young woman, as to be described as a 'breast mouse'. Fibroadenomata are not always well encapsulated or mobile and at biopsy may be found to be ill defined – forming a diffuse area of fibroadenomatoid hyperplasia.

Some are comprised almost completely of epithelial tissue and may grow to quite a large size. These large, soft fibroadenomas are sometimes known as cystosarcoma phylloides, Brodie's tumour or giant fibroadenoma. Such tumours have a tendency to recur locally and either the epithelial or stromal elements have the potential for malignant change, forming a carcinoma or sarcoma respectively.

Benign soft tissue tumours.   These are a heterogeneous group of tumours derived from the breast stroma and the commonest is the lipoma.

Circumscribed lipomas may be found in the breast and give the physical signs of a smooth mobile swelling which may be mistaken for a cyst. Ill-defined lipomata occur commonly in the axilla and invariably they contain islands of breast tissue.

Intramammary lymph nodes are sometimes palpable clinically and often seen on mammograms and they probably represent lymphoid hyperplasia in response to some undetected stimulus within the breast or else they are part of a generalized lymphoid hyperplasia.

Carcinoma of the breast

The clinical features associated with carcinoma of the breast can be considerable and diverse. The local features in the breast have already been alluded to in earlier parts of this Chapter, but it is important to remember that carcinoma of the breast is not a single entity. It is a group of diseases which have the common factor of a primary tumour arising within the breast. The progress of that tumour within the breast and the pattern of its spread to adjacent tissues, to regional lymph nodes and to the rest of the body can vary considerably. This variation is in part related to the histological type of the primary tumour, but it is also related to other biological features which are, even now, ill understood.

For example, we are all aware of women who present with a 2 cm mass in the outer half of the breast which is not associated with any palpable nodes and yet who die within 6–12 months of mastectomy with widespread metastases in lung, pleura, liver and bone. On the other hand, a similar woman with a similar tumour and a similar history may proceed to mastectomy and live for 20 or 30 years with only slowly progressive metastatic disease at one site. The skin is a common site for metastatic disease which does not always progress rapidly.

The different biological features of breast cancer behaviour remain a challenge not only to the therapist but also the laboratory worker since attempts should continue to be made to predict the prognostic behaviour of any one particular tumour in any one particular patient.

The features of disseminated disease lie outside the scope of this Chapter and this book, and it would be better to concentrate on the local situation in the breast.

The commonest presentation of breast carcinoma is of a lump in the breast found by the patient herself. This may be the result of regular self-examination or it may be the result of an accidental examination whilst washing or because of local pain or tenderness. The size of a tumour felt by the patient is not commonly less than 1 cm, although in fortunate occasions, patients can detect 0.5 cm masses in breasts which are otherwise soft and absolutely normal. As already mentioned, the ability to feel a hard swelling in the breast depends on the consistency of the surrounding breast tissue and it is easier to feel a tumour in a soft fatty breast than it is in a firm, dysplastic breast.

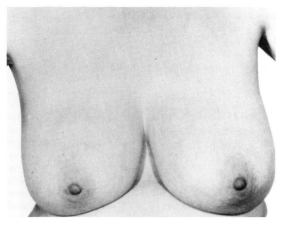
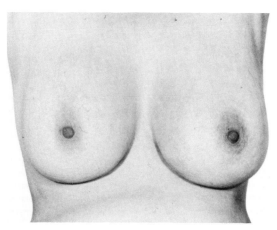

Fig. 2.13 This woman has a palpable tumour in her right breast. On inspection, the left breast is a little larger than the right although the tumour is not seen. (a) Arms down, (b) arms elevated.

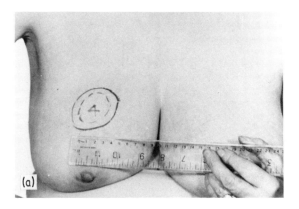

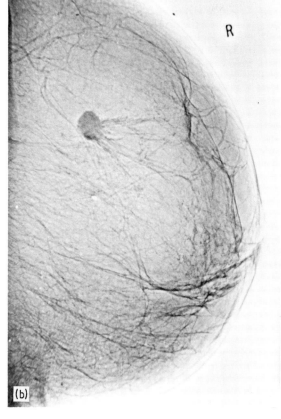

Fig. 2.14 (a) The tumour in the upper half of the right breast measures 4 cm. (b) The xeromammogram (lateral projection) shows the tumour mass to be less than 2 cm (compare with the nipple) but it has anterior spiculations.

The size of the tumour felt will often be larger than the pathological or radiological size of the tumour which is seen on mammography and removed for pathology (Figs 2.13 and 2.14). This phenomenon of the clinical overestimation of the size of a breast tumour was reported by Leborgne (1951) and it is sometimes known in the radiological literature as 'Leborgne's Law'.

Fig. 2.15 demonstrates the correlation between clinical measurement of size, radiological measurement of size on film mammography and pathological measurement of tumour size made in the laboratory at the time of tumour biopsy. These figures were taken from a series of 100 breast tumours removed at the Royal Marsden in the years 1960–65. It shows the regular clinical overestimation of the size of the tumour, particularly as the tumours increase in size. The irregular nature of many tumours' edges makes accurate measurement difficult but this may in part account for the difference between the clinical, radiograph and pathological measurements. It is possible also that there is an increased vascularity or stromal response at the periphery of many tumours which does not produce much histological abnormality but which does produce a palpable thickening.

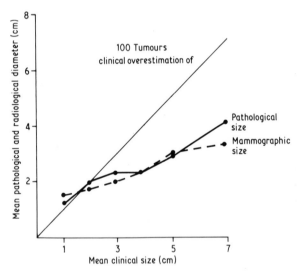

Fig. 2.15   This graph shows the close relationship between the pathological and radiological measurements of tumour size compared with the clinical size which is usually greater (from 100 cases treated surgically after clinical examination and film mammography at Royal Marsden Hospital, 1965–71). (Toussis and Greening, unpublished communication).

The increasing size of a breast tumour – regardless of its pathological type or grade – is related to an increased mortality (Fig. 2.16). Many workers have described the decreasing prognosis related to increase in size and of course this forms one of the major features of the TNM staging system (see Chapter 11).

The closer correlation between radiological and pathological size

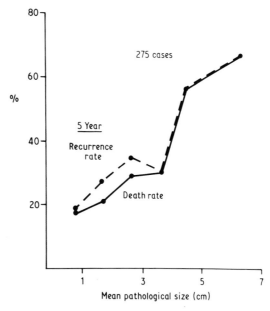

Fig. 2.16 This graph shows the increase in 5-year mortality (and recurrence) associated with increase in the pathological diameter of the tumour (follow-up of 275 cases treated at Royal Marsden Hospital between 1960 and 1965).

encouraged the TNM Committee of the International Union against Cancer to recommend the use of mammographic tumour measurement in preference to clinical tumour measurement in 1974 (UICC, 1974 and 1978).

In situ carcinoma

The clinical features of non-invasive carcinoma are often those of the associated dysplasia in which the tumour is detected only by histological examination. The smallest microscopic, non-infiltrating tumours are found almost as a histological accident in the careful assessment of biopsy material. The indications for the biopsy may be clinical – a lump or firm area of nodularity in the breast – or radiological, associated with localized calcification. In an analysis of 30 cases of non-invasive intraduct carcinoma treated at the Royal Marsden Hospital, Millis and Thynne (1975) showed that 50% of the cases had a palpable mass greater than 2 cm in size. Clinical examination suggested that this was a localized area of benign breast disease but it was not possible to exclude malignancy.

In situ disease detected by mammography may be impalpable and some method of localization is needed prior to biopsy (see Chapter 7). The prognosis of the patient and her residual breast tissue after the detection and diagnosis of non-infiltrating carcinoma – and especially lobular carcinoma *in situ* – is such a variable situation that management can vary from continuing careful observation on the one hand to more extensive surgery up to and including a modified radical mastectomy with a simultaneous, mirror image biopsy of the opposite breast. The decision to biopsy the opposite breast is made more frequently in the presence of lobular carcinoma *in situ* than with ductal carcinoma *in situ* and the site of the biopsy may be a mirror image if there are no other clinical or radiological areas of suspicion at different sites in the apparently unaffected breast.

Infiltrating carcinoma

The majority of infiltrating carcinomas have an associated fibroblastic or fibrous stroma ('scirrhous') and they may be associated with evidence of multifocal origin and areas of non-infiltrating duct carcinoma. These comprise 70–80% of most breast carcinomas and they give rise to the clinical physical signs which are related to the size and extent of the tumour within the breast.

Primary tumour size

This forms the basis for staging the extent of the tumour according to the TNM system. Increase in size of the tumour is usually associated with a worse prognosis and with involvement of other structures such as the skin with formation of dimples because of infiltration of the ligaments of Astley-Cooper with contractile fibrous tissue (Figs 2.5 and 2.6).

If the tumour extends deeply and is tethered to the pectoral fascia this can be detected by assessing the mobility of the tumour in two directions when pectoralis major is lax and when it is contracted by asking the patient to push her hands against her hip. Further deep extension of the tumour into the chest wall is a very advanced sign as is direct involvement of the skin (Fig. 2.8). Another secondary sign of advanced local disease is the presence of cutaneous oedema (peau d'orange) (Fig. 2.7). This is related to lymphatic stasis, either because of the adjacent primary tumour or because of lymph node stasis in the axilla. In the latter case the oedema is first seen in the infra-areolar portion of the breast.

Peau d'orange and erythema of the skin are signs of recent and rapid progression and they are usually regarded as signs of inoperability because of the grave risk of local recurrence in the operation area.

Denoix (1970) has described rapidly growing tumours ('poussée evolutif') and the most severe form of this is the so-called 'inflammatory carcinoma'.

Some rapidly-progressive tumours occur during pregnancy and lactation (Fig. 2.17) and, when this occurs, the prognosis will be grave. The physiological changes in the breast related to pregnancy often lead to a delay in diagnosis and this may contribute to a worse prognosis in addition to the high histological grade of the tumours seen in pregnancy. In

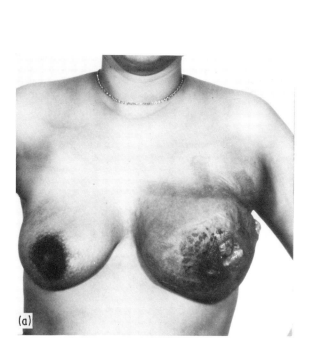
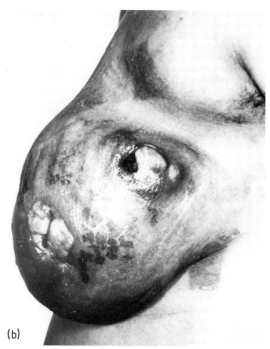

Fig. 2.17   This young woman developed an 'abscess' in the eighth month of pregnancy. Two biopsies were made adjacent to the nipple (a) – note the pigmentation of the normal nipple and in the upper outer quadrant (b). Neither has healed and the tumour is fungating through the wounds.

particular, the prognosis is worst when the diagnosis is made and treatment started in the second half of pregnancy (Peters, 1968).

The slow and insidious rate of growth of other breast tumours has been mentioned and such cancers will often carry a much better prognosis, and women with such tumours will commonly delay in presenting for medical advice.

Patey and Scarff (1928) described a histological method of grading the malignancy of a breast carcinoma: Bloom and Richardson (1957) reported the application of this grading system to a large series of patients at the Middlesex Hospital. They were able to show that grade was related to prognosis and Table 2.1 illustrates that very clearly.

Table 2.1

Grade	Cases	Per cent	5 yr mortality
I	363	26%	20%
II	640	45%	50%
III	408	29%	65%

Progression of an infiltrating tumour within the breast is associated with an increasing degree of spread to the regional lymph nodes and in the bloodstream to produce distant metastases.

Regional lymph node disease.   Clinical examination of the axilla is not a very reliable indicator of axillary nodal pathology and unfortunately an inaccuracy of 25–30% in the clinical assessment of involvement of axillary lymph nodes is well recognized and demonstrated in Tables 2.2 and 2.3.

Table 2.2   Showing the correlation between clinical examination of the axilla and the pathological examination of the lymph nodes in 672 cases of breast carcinoma treated at the Royal Marsden Hospital (1945–59).

Clinical		Pathologies			Agreement
		Total	Negative	Positive	
Impalpable	(N0)	313	188	125	60%
Palpable and mobile	(N1)	306	61	245	80%
Palpable and fixed	(N2)	53	2	51	96%

Table 2.3   Showing the correlation between clinical and pathological assessment of axillary lymph nodes and including an assessment of the contralateral axilla (Cutler, 1969).

Clinical		Pathological	
Ipsilateral	Contralateral	Negative	Positive
Not palpable	Not palpable	754	448
Palpable	Not palpable	158	302
Palpable	Palpable	39*	46
		21% Palpable Ipsilateral nodes	56% Impalpable Ipsilateral nodes

*This small group has best (81%) 10 yr survival (Cutler *et al.*, 1969).

As well as its relation to decreased survival, increasing tumour size is related to increasing degree of lymph node involvement (Robbins, 1962) (Table 2.4).

It has been shown that for any given tumour size, the association of skin tethering increases the likelihood of axillary lymph node involvement (Melville, unpublished communication).

The internal mammary lymph node chain is an important pathological route of spread of breast carcinomas – particularly those which are situated in the centre and inner half of the breast (Handley, 1972). The nodes in it

Table 2.4 (From the Memorial Hospital, New York.) Shows the relationship between increasing tumour size ((a) for tumours which are less than 2 cm in diameter, (b) for tumours of 2–2.9 cm and (c) for tumours of 4–4.9 cm), pathological involvement of the axilla from lowest (level I) to highest or apical nodes (level III) and survival over 5, 10 and 15 years (Robbins, 1962).

		5 yr (%)	10 yr (%)	15 yr (%)
(a)	Lesion < 2 cm			
	Negative nodes	87	68	59
	Level I	73	63	50
	Level II	76	65	59
	Level III	46	26	18
(b)	Lesion 2–2.9 cm			
	Negative nodes	72	52	35
	Level I	70	52	44
	Level II	44	32	19
	Level III	44	24	14
(c)	Lesion 4–4.9 cm			
	Negative nodes	60	38	30
	Level I	53	32	21
	Level II	41	18	12
	Level III	28	15	10

are small and because of their anatomical site, they do not lend themselves to clinical assessment and only rarely present with detectable, anteriorly extending, deposits.

Metastatic disease.   The outcome for most patients with a diagnosis of breast cancer is determined by the extent of blood-borne spread before diagnosis and before primary treatment.

The aim for the earlier diagnosis of primary breast carcinoma is the detection of an increasing number of tumours which are localized to the breast.

The methods of diagnosis of disseminated disease lie outside the scope of this book, but the careful surgeon, physician or radiotherapist will always attempt to make some staging assessment of the extent of spread of the tumour before making any final decisions on definitive therapy.

It remains fundamental that we treat patients according to an accurate estimate of the stage of disease, rather than, for example, operating on a woman's left breast and removing it as a matter of urgency before proper thought has been given to the possibility of distant spread.

Secondary tumours in the breast

Metastatic carcinoma, melanoma and lymphoma have all been described in the breast and the method of presentation is usually that of a lump (or lumps) found by the patient or seen on routine mammography.

Sarcomas

Malignant mesothelial or connective tissue tumours can arise *de novo* within the breast or from pre-existing benign tumours such as fibroadenomas.

A fibrosarcoma or stromal cell sarcoma is the commonest soft tissue tumour reported, although malignant fibrous histiocytoma has recently been described in the breast.

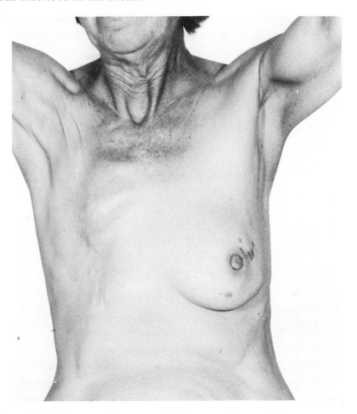

Fig. 2.18   This woman has a second primary carcinoma with cutaneous metastases in the left breast more than ten years after a successful right radical mastectomy.

These tumours present as a lump requiring excisional biopsy for diagnosis and usually needing a total mastectomy to achieve local control and to avoid local recurrence. Axillary lymph node invasion is rare, and pulmonary metastases are the common demonstration of dissemination.

Haemangiolymphangio-sarcomas have been described in the oedematous, postmastectomy arm (Stewart and Treves, 1948).

Radiation-induced osteosarcomas of soft tissue and of the shoulder girdle and radiation-induced fibrosarcomas have been reported within the treatment area following postmastectomy irradiation.

These are rare conditions which are occasionally seen in the follow-up examinations of women treated for breast cancer.

Carcinoma of the second breast

Women who have had treatment for one breast cancer are at risk for the development of a second primary carcinoma and clinical examination of the remaining breast and regular mammography play an important part in the detection of second, metachronous tumours.

Fig. 2.18 shows a woman who has a second primary tumour with rapidly-progressive cutaneous deposits appearing more than ten years after an otherwise successful right radical mastectomy.

Synchronous bilateral primary tumours are seen in less than 5% of cases and, as already mentioned, more frequently in young women with a family history.

EAST GLAMORGAN HOSPITAL.
CHURCH VILLAGE. near PONTYPRIDD

3 MAMMOGRAPHIC TECHNIQUE

Olivia L. Wilson

It is not difficult to radiograph breast tissue. However, it does require a degree of application in order to produce high quality images of the complete breast regularly.

The radiographic techniques described aim to provide the radiologist with mammograms in which the breast is well-positioned and the images sufficiently detailed to enable subtle differences in the soft tissues to be recognized. In addition, where treatment is needed, the aim is to provide the surgeon or radiotherapist with precise information regarding the size and position of abnormalities.

An important aspect of mammographic technique is concerned with the general approach to the patient. Most patients are tense and afraid of the investigative procedures and the possible findings. In addition, many patients are embarassed by the techniques used to obtain the best images. Patients may assume awkward or defensive postures, be distracted or distant and appear not to hear instructions. It is essential to communicate with the patient in order to give reassurance and obtain relaxation of the shoulders. Most patients will need to be reminded to relax their shoulders two or three times during each view in order to obtain the correct positioning. The procedures should be explained where possible, especially where they are likely to be uncomfortable and essential to the radiographic result. The radiographer should never be tentative, even when inexperienced in mammography. A firm approach to positioning the patient should be combined with a sympathetic attitude. The radiographer who appears assured and friendly and takes the trouble to talk the patient through the procedures will obtain the desired results: a more responsive, relaxed patient and better mammograms.

SELECTION OF APPROPRIATE VIEWS

Patients for mammography fall into two categories. The first category consists of patients presenting for screening examination. The examination of choice here is the supine medio-lateral technique. This view fulfills all the requirements for an ideal screening examination: sensitivity, a low patient dose, the ability to be reproduced at follow-up examinations and the maximum amount of information in a single view for economy. The erect oblique technique may also be used as a screening examination.

The second category consists of patients presenting with symptoms, clinical abnormalities or previous history of breast pathology. These patients require a more definitive examination in order to indicate precisely the position, size and nature of the abnormality. The basic mammographic examination for these patients consists of a lateral view and a cranio-caudad view. The lateral view may be taken either supine or erect. The supine medio-lateral technique may be used for all patients. It is useful for patients with small dense breasts and particularly for patients with silicone implants, where the area between the implant and the rib cage can be difficult to demonstrate. In addition, it is the easiest technique to use with patients who have had wide excisional surgery or radiotherapy. The erect medio-lateral technique may be used for all patients, but is usually less successful than the supine medio-lateral for patients with very small breasts unless sponge wedges are employed. Patients with a depressed sternum or kyphosis will be more easily positioned by the erect latero-medial technique. This may also produce images with greater detail of abnormalities which are medially placed. Extended cranio-caudad views may be useful as a supplement to the standard cranio-caudad. They may be used for patients with large breasts where the tissues cannot be included in one image. In addition, the extended cranio-caudad techniques may be used to give added information on abnormalities close to the lateral or medial border of the breast. A further supplementary technique which may be useful either for patients with large breasts or for demonstrating the axillary tail is the axillary tail oblique technique. The axillary tail oblique view will often show axillary nodes, but if a more comprehensive view is required, a true axillary projection must be used. The erect axillary is the technique of choice as the axillary nodes are less likely to be obscured by the scapula or shoulder girdle than in the supine view. However, the supine axillary technique is useful for patients who are infirm or short of breath and find it difficult to maintain the necessary position during the long exposure time required for axillary views. In addition, patients who are very obese may be more easily positioned by this technique.

TECHNIQUES

The following descriptions of technique are for patients of average size. Patients outside the normal range may require some modification of the method and consequently the results obtained may differ from the ideal. In addition, some minor differences in technique will be necessary when using xerographic plates instead of radiographic film. In particular, it is important to remember, when using xerographic plates, that the image area does not coincide with that of the cassette.

The supine medio-lateral view

The patient lies supine on the couch with the arm on the side under examination extended 100° to the body and the hand on the pillow beside the head. Cassettes containing xerographic plates should be placed in a large tunnel and positioned at an angle so that the top of the cassette is beneath the patient's shoulder, and the leading edge of the lower half of the cassette remains visible. Cassettes containing radiographic film should be positioned at an angle with the top corner touching the ribs at the axillary tail.

A sponge wedge is selected which has a thick edge approximately corresponding to the depth of rib cage between the lateral edge of the breast and the cassette (Fig. 3.1). The thick edge is placed against the ribs with the top of the wedge in the axilla, and held firmly while the patient rolls slowly and smoothly on to their side. The position of the hips is adjusted at this stage until the patient feels steady. The patient is rolled slightly further until the breast tissue falls away from the ribs. One hand is placed under the lateral side of the breast in order to check that the sponge is still in position in the axilla. The hand is then withdrawn, smoothing any creases in the skin at the same time.

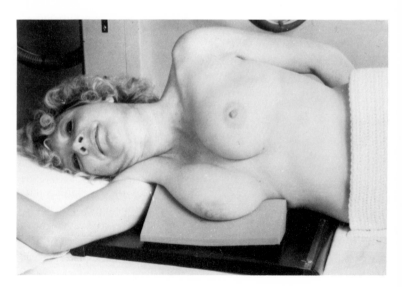

Fig. 3.1   The supine medio-lateral technique: position of the patient prior to the application of compression.

The cone is angled 10° to the body, centred and rotated so that the whole of the breast will be included in the final image. The cone is moved into position against the ribs one inch to the raised side of the midline, whilst holding the other breast out of the way. Compression is applied until the breast is firmly held and an even thickness throughout (Fig. 3.2). It is important to keep the cone pushed well into the ribs and to ensure that the patient does not roll backward from the correct position.

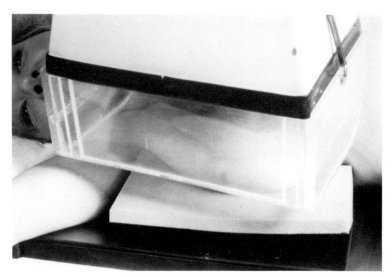

Fig. 3.2   The supine medio-lateral technique: patient positioned and compression applied.

The correct technique should show all the breast tissue with the nipple in profile and include the retromammary space and part of the axilla (Fig. 3.3).

The erect medio-lateral view

The patient stands or is seated facing the equipment which is set for laterally positioned techniques. The patient's hand on the side under examination is positioned holding the mid-point of the back edge of the cassette. The patient is turned 45° away from the cassette, and positioned so that the leading edge of the cassette, although not in contact with the patient, will be located behind the lateral margin of the breast when it is brought forward. The lower edge of the cassette is positioned so that it will be located one inch below the inframammary crease. A laterally placed sponge wedge may be positioned at this stage.

The upper outer quadrant of the breast is grasped firmly between the thumb and fingers and is lifted and pulled forward whilst simultaneously bringing the patient's side into contact with the cassette. The patient is

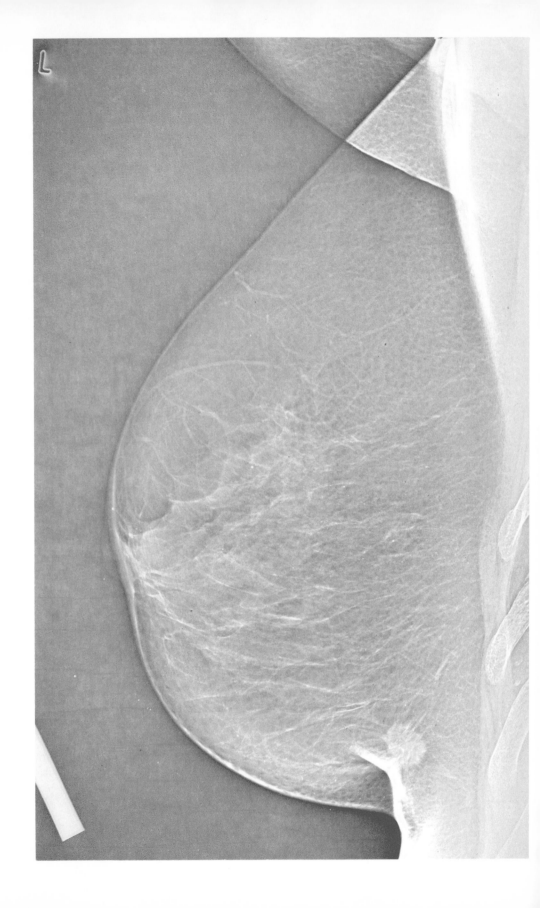

twisted until the lateral side of the breast is pressed against the cassette. This procedure ensures that the most lateral part of the breast is included in the image. The breast is pulled firmly up and forward from the ribs with the fingers spread in an arc over the lower medial area of the breast. A medially placed sponge wedge may be positioned at this stage. Compression should be applied until the breast tissue is an even thickness throughout (Fig. 3.4). The supporting hand may be gradually withdrawn as the compression holds the breast firmly in position.

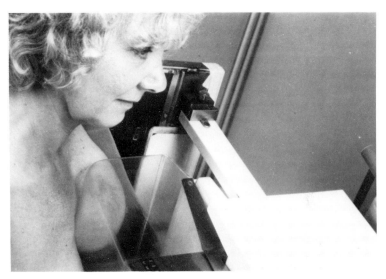

Fig. 3.4   The erect medio-lateral technique: patient positioned and compression applied.

The correct technique should show all the breast tissue with the nipple in profile and either the ends of the ribs or the pectoral muscle visible at the base of the breast (Fig. 3.5).

The erect latero-medial view

The patient stands or is seated facing the equipment which is set for laterally positioned techniques. The arm on the side under examination is raised to shoulder height and rested on a suitable surface. A medially placed sponge wedge may be positioned at this stage. The patient is moved forward so that the edge of the cassette is between the breasts. The breast is pulled firmly up and forward from the ribs with the fingers spread in an arc over the lower lateral area of the breast. The patient is rotated toward

Fig. 3.3   The supine medio-lateral technique: xeromammogram, negative mode.

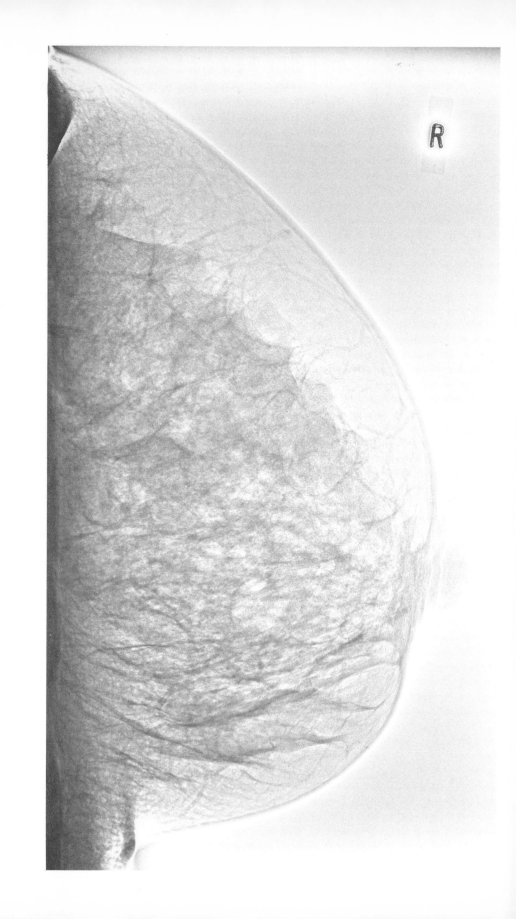

the equipment so that compression may be started at the extreme lateral margin. A laterally placed sponge wedge may be positioned at this stage. Compression should be applied until the breast is an even thickness throughout. The supporting hand may be gradually withdrawn as the compression holds the breast more firmly in position.

The correct technique should show all the breast tissue with either the ends of the ribs or the pectoral muscle visible at the base of the breast. The nipple may not be in profile in patients with a normal rib cage if compression is started at the extreme lateral margin of the breast as recommended (Fig. 3.6).

The cranio-caudad view

The patient stands or is seated facing the equipment which is set for cranio-caudadly positioned techniques. The arm on the side under examination is extended in front of the patient with the hand holding an appropriate part of the equipment. The patient is turned 30° away from the cassette. The patient should not be in contact with the cassette at this stage. A sponge wedge may be positioned if required. The breast is raised and supported with the fingers together at the inframammary crease. The patient is brought forward until the rib cage is just in contact with the edge of the cassette, which is raised until opposite the inframammary crease. Areas of the breast may be excluded from the image following compression if the cassette is either higher or lower than this position. The fingers are withdrawn from beneath the breast, gently pulling the breast tissue towards the nipple. The skin above the breast is pulled toward the nipple and held firmly in position.

The patient is turned approximately 20° toward the cassette, ensuring that the lateral part of the breast remains within the image area. The patient is then instructed to lean slightly forward and compression of the breast is commenced. Once the central and lateral areas of the breast are held in position by the compression cone, but without being fully compressed, the patient is encouraged to push the head as far forward around the cone as possible (Fig. 3.7). This procedure ensures that the medial area of the breast is brought fully over the image area. Further compression is applied until the breast is firmly held and an even thickness throughout. The hand holding the breast may be gradually withdrawn as the compression holds the breast more firmly in position.

The correct technique should show the maximum amount of breast tissue with the nipple in profile (Fig. 3.8). It is not possible to include the axillary tail in a cranio-caudad view.

Fig. 3.5   The erect medio-lateral technique: xeromammogram, positive mode.

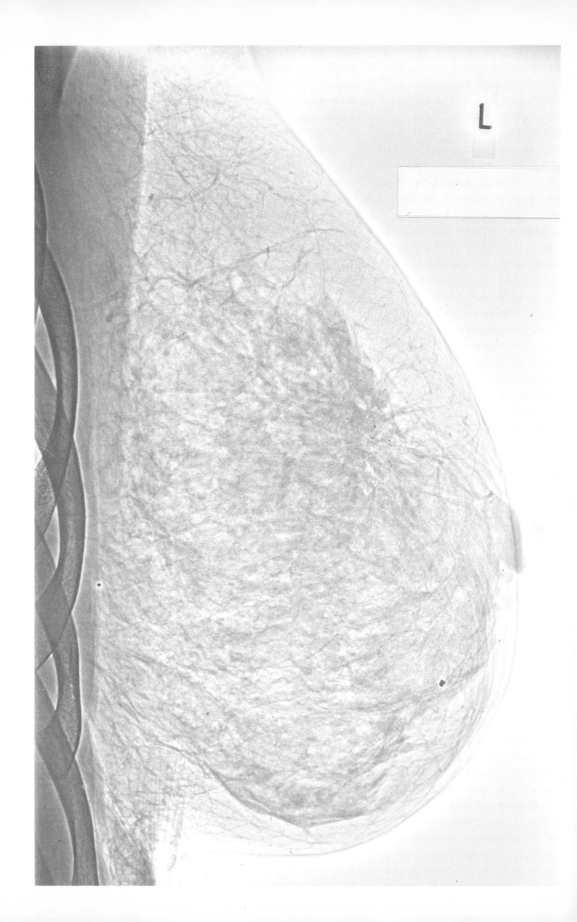

Fig. 3.6   The erect latero-medial
technique: xeromammogram, positive
mode.

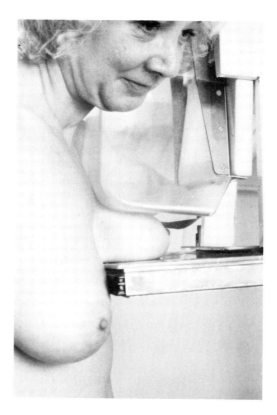

Fig. 3.7   The cranio-caudad
technique: patient positioned and
compression applied. ▶

Fig. 3.8   The cranio-caudad
technique: xeromammogram, positive
mode. ▼

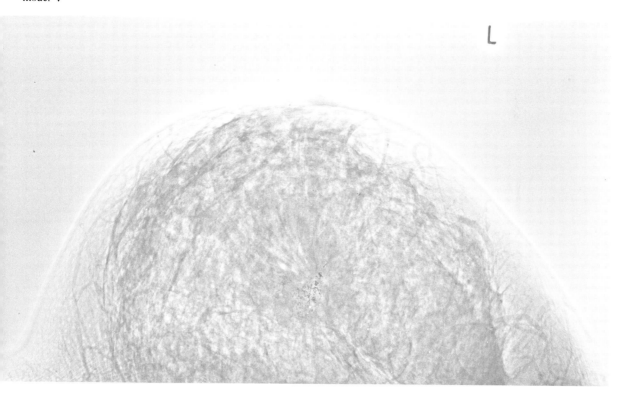

The extended cranio-caudad views

Lateral extension

The patient stands or is seated facing the equipment which is set for cranio-caudally positioned techniques. The hand and forearm on the side under examination are rested on the edge of the cassette to one side. The patient is turned approximately 60° away from the cassette so that only the lateral side of the breast is presented to the front edge of the cassette. The patient's side should not be in contact with the cassette at this stage. The lateral part of the breast is lifted and supported with the fingers together to the level of the upper end of the inframammary crease. The patient is brought forward until the rib cage is just in contact with the edge of the cassette, which is raised until opposite the upper end of the inframammary crease. The medial part of the breast is not included in the image. It is necessary to move the arm further forward at this stage and instruct the patient to lean slightly toward the side under examination. With the shoulder completely relaxed, the skin just below the shoulder joint is pulled down and forward whilst compression is applied. The hand holding the breast may be gradually withdrawn as the compression holds the breast more firmly in position. The compression which may be applied is usually less than that which can be achieved on the standard cranio-caudad view and some compensation in exposure may be required.

The correct technique should show the whole of the lateral area of the breast and most of the central area, with the nipple in profile (Fig. 3.9).

Medial extension

The patient stands or is seated facing the equipment which is set for cranio-caudadly positioned techniques. The arm on the side under examination is extended in front of the patient with the hand holding an appropriate part of the machine. The patient is positioned facing the equipment, but it is sometimes necessary to turn the head away from the side under examination when using certain types of equipment. The patient is aligned with the cassette so that the medial quadrant of the side under examination and part of the medial quadrant of the other side will be included in the image. The patient should not be in contact with the cassette at this stage. A sponge wedge may be positioned if required.

The medial quadrants of both breasts are raised and supported with the fingers together at the inframammary crease. The patient is brought forward until the rib cage is in contact with the cassette, which is raised until opposite the inframammary crease. The fingers are withdrawn from beneath the breast, gently pulling the breast tissue towards the nipple. The skin over the sternum is pulled down very firmly and held in position. The patient is instructed to lean toward the equipment as far as possible whilst rotating both shoulders anteriorly. Compression is then applied from just below the sterno–clavicular joints. The hand holding the breasts

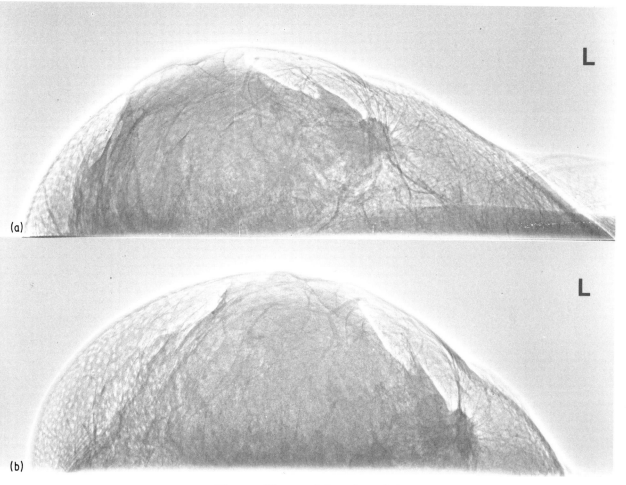

(a)

(b)

L

L

Fig. 3.9   The extended cranio-caudad technique, lateral extension (a) and the standard cranio-caudad technique (b): comparative xeromammograms.

may be gradually withdrawn as the compression holds them more firmly in position. The degree of compression which can be applied is usually less than that which can be achieved on the cranio-caudad view and some compensation in exposure may be required.

The correct technique should show the whole of the medial part of the breast under examination and part of the medial area of the other breast (Fig. 3.10).

The oblique view

The equipment is set at an angle between 30° and 45° to the lateral position. Patients with small breasts are usually positioned more easily at 30° and those with large breasts at 45° away from the cassette. The patient

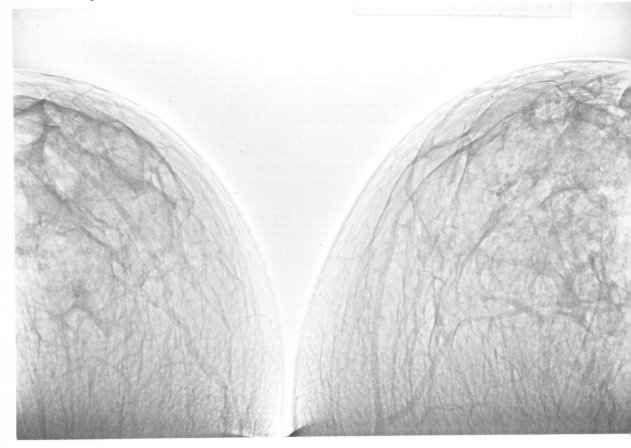

Fig. 3.10   The extended cranio-caudad technique, medial extension:
xeromammogram, positive mode.

stands or is seated facing the equipment and is turned 45° away from the
cassette. The upper arm on the side under examination is rested on the
upper edge of the cassette when using radiographic film. The upper arm is
positioned in front of the upper part of the cassette when using xerographic
plates. The patient's elbow is bent at 90° and the hand supported on a suitable surface. The patient is positioned so that the leading edge of the
cassette, although not in contact with the patient, will be located behind the
lateral margin of the breast when the patient is brought forward. The lower
edge of the cassette is positioned so that it will be located one inch below the
inframammary crease. A laterally placed sponge wedge may be positioned
at this stage.

The upper outer quadrant of the breast is grasped firmly between the
thumb and fingers, and is lifted and pulled forward whilst simultaneously
bringing the patient's side into contact with the cassette. The patient is
twisted until the lateral side of the breast is pressed against the cassette,

ensuring that the patient's side remains against the edge of the cassette. The breast is pushed firmly up and forward from the ribs with the flat of the hand. This is best achieved from beneath the breast by crouching in front of the patient. Folds of abdominal fat should be removed from the image area at this stage by adjusting the position of the patient's hips. A medially placed sponge wedge may be positioned if required. Compression should be applied until the breast tissue is firmly held and an even thickness throughout (Fig. 3.11). The patient is instructed to hold the other breast out of the way if necessary. The supporting hand may be gradually withdrawn as the compression holds the breast more firmly in position. The skin of the side of the rib cage should be pulled backwards gently from the behind to remove any folds at the lateral margin of the breast.

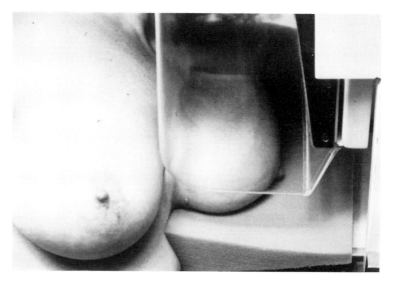

Fig. 3.11   The oblique technique: patient positioned and compression applied.

The correct technique should show all the breast tissue with the nipple in profile and either the ends of the ribs or the pectoral muscle visible at the base of the breast (Fig. 3.12).

The axillary tail oblique

The equipment is set as for the standard oblique technique and the patient is initially positioned in a similar manner so that the leading edge of the cassette, although not in contact with the patient, will be located behind the lateral margin of the breast when the patient is brought forward. However, the upper edge of the cassette is positioned so that it will be located against the patient's back just below the shoulder joint.

The tissue of the axillary tail is grasped firmly between the thumb and

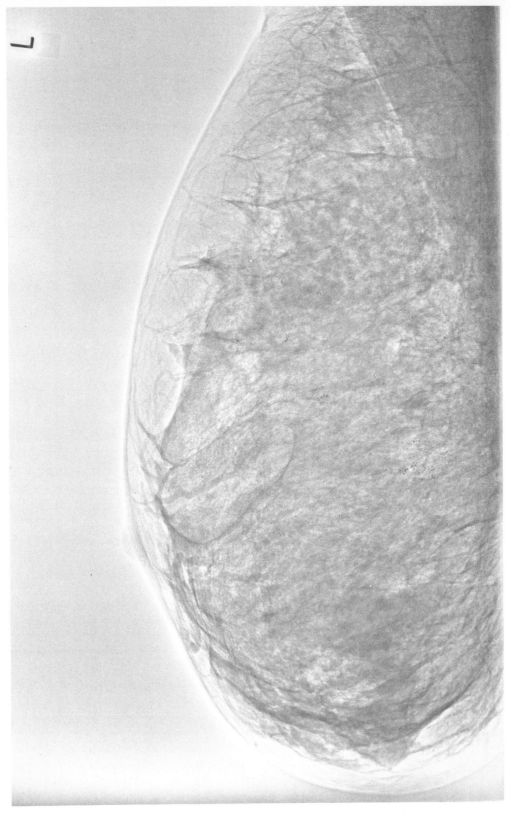

▲ Fig. 3.12 The oblique technique: xeromammogram, positive mode.

Fig. 3.13 The axillary tail oblique: xeromammogram. ▶

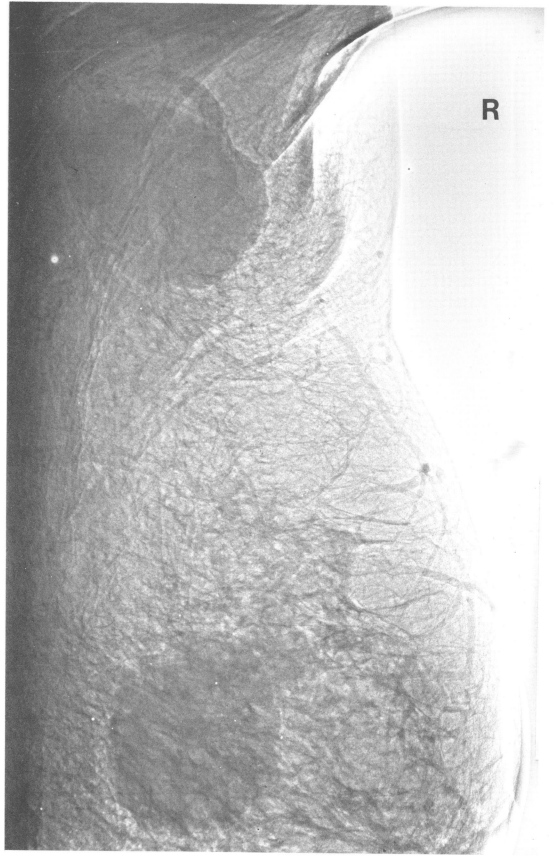

R

fingers and is lifted and pulled forward whilst simultaneously bringing the patient's side into contact with the cassette. It is necessary to move the arm further forward at this stage and instruct the patient to lean slightly toward the side under examination. The remainder of the technique is the same as that described for the standard oblique view, except that the patient should not be twisted toward the cassette to the same degree.

The correct technique should show all of the axillary tail and most of the axilla (Fig. 3.13).

The erect axillary view

The patient stands or is seated facing the equipment which is set for laterally positioned techniques. The patient is turned 90° away from the cassette. The equipment should be positioned so that the upper edge of the cassette is level with the top of the shoulder joint. The compression cone is retracted to its fullest extent. The arm on the side under examination is extended across the front of the cassette. The elbow is bent so that the upper arm forms an angle of 45° to the rib cage with the hand holding an

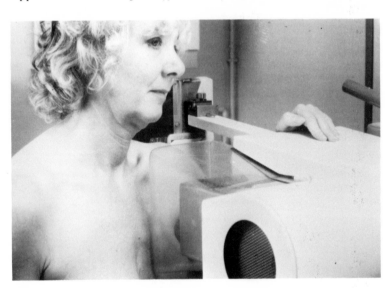

Fig. 3.14   The erect axillary technique: patient positioned.

appropriate part of the equipment. The patient is instructed to lean slightly forward, rotating the shoulder joint anteriorally. The patient is moved sideways until the axilla is positioned in front of the cassette. The patient is instructed to relax the shoulder and is rotated until the scapula is pressed flat against the cassette. Compression is not applied (Fig. 3.14).

The correct technique should show the axilla fully. The major part of the shoulder joint and some of the rib cage will be included in the image (Fig. 3.15).

Fig. 3.15   The erect axillary technique: xeromammogram. ▶

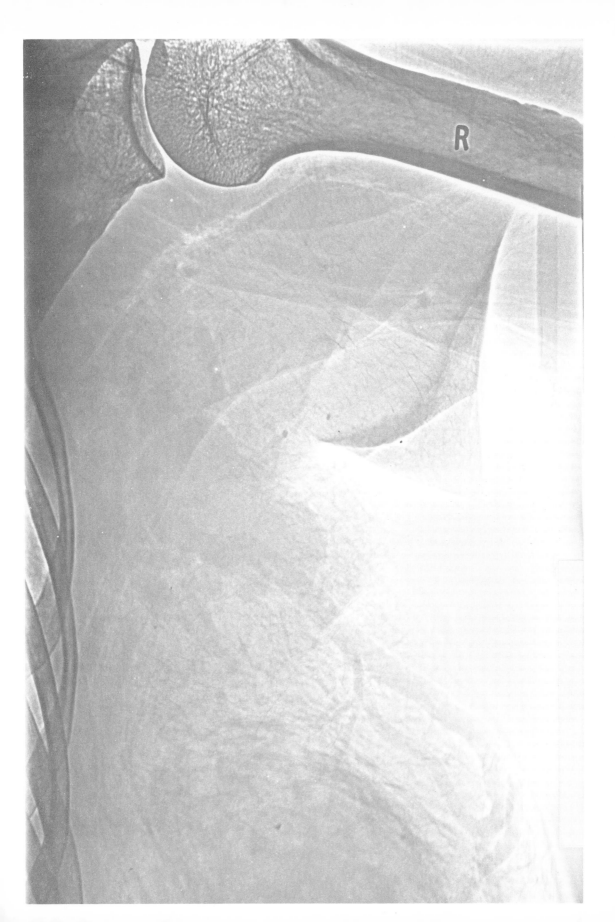

The supine axillary view

The patient lies supine on the couch with the upper arm on the side under examination forming an angle of 45° to the body and the hand on the pillow. The cassette is placed with the upper edge level with the top of the shoulder joint and the axilla positioned centrally. The patient is rolled towards the side under examination until the scapula is pressed flat against the cassette. The cone is centred directly over the axilla. Compression is not applied (Fig. 3.16).

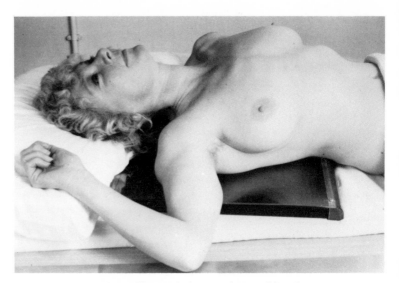

Fig. 3.16   The supine axillary technique: patient positioned.

The correct technique should show all of the axilla. The major part of the shoulder joint and some of the rib cage will be included in the image (Fig. 3.17).

THE USE OF SPONGE WEDGES

Wedges of fine mammographic sponge are a useful aid in many mammographic techniques. They may be used to support and maintain the correct position of the breast. However, the main advantage of using sponge wedges is that better compression may be achieved. Many patients

Fig. 3.17   The supine axillary technique: xeromammogram.

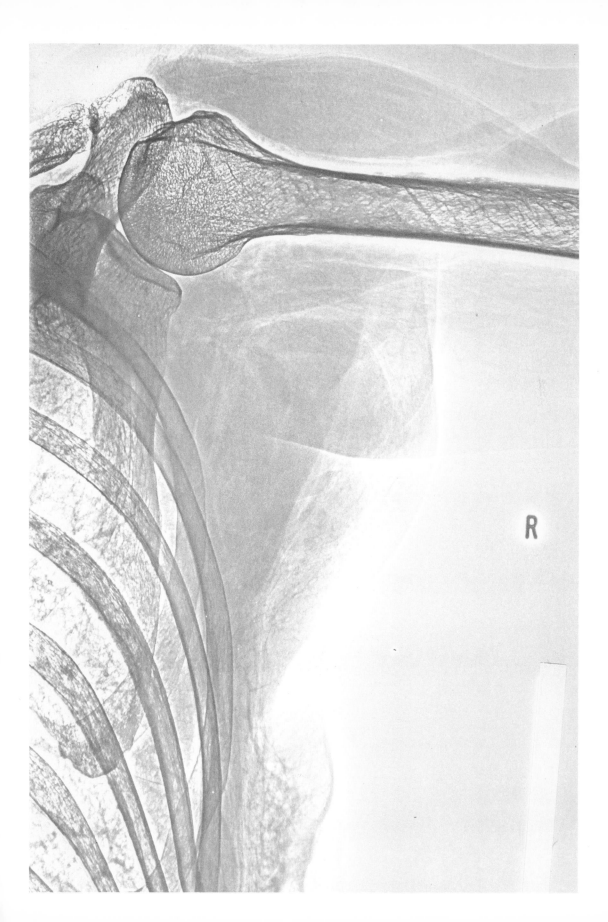

R

tolerate greater compression when cushioned by sponges, and a more uniform thickness of breast tissue may be obtained.

A laterally placed sponge wedge is always used in the supine medio-lateral technique. Sponges may be used laterally in erect lateral techniques, in which case the thin edge of the wedge should be towards the base of the breast overlapping the edge of the cassette. A small sponge wedge may be used in the cranio-caudad technique, in which case the thick end of the wedge should be towards the base of the breast and the longest side uppermost. A laterally placed sponge wedge may be used for the oblique views, the thick end of the wedge should be towards the base of the breast and the top well into the axilla. Medially placed sponges may be used in erect lateral and oblique techniques where a patient has small breasts or a prominent sternum.

LOCALIZATION TECHNIQUES

Localization techniques are used to identify the precise position of impalpable lesions for cytology or biopsy. In addition, the same techniques may be used to provide images in which selected areas are shown in greater detail.

Technique

Mammograms are selected which demonstrate the abnormality in two planes, and the position of the abnormality is defined by two measurements on each view. A perpendicular line is drawn from the base of the breast to the nipple. The distance between the nipple and the level of the abnormality is measured along this line. The distance between the perpendicular and the abnormality is also measured. For example, an abnormality might be recorded as: 3 cm behind and 2 cm above the nipple in the lateral view, 3 cm behind the nipple and 4 cm medial to the nipple in the cranio-caudad view.

The initial localization procedure is aimed at providing images approximately 10 cm in diameter. The patient is positioned as for the original standard view, but without compression. Compression is simulated with a plastic ruler, the recorded distances are measured and the position of the abnormality marked with a felt tip pen. The patient and the equipment are carefully positioned so that the mark is directly over the centre of the image area. The breast must be held very firmly in place whilst the compression is applied. The same technique is used to provide a localized version of the standard view in the second plane.

Where the abnormality is in the centre of the image on both localization views, and is shown in sufficient detail, further techniques may not be required. However, if the abnormality is not central or if more accurate localization is required, further techniques may be used to provide images approximately 5 cm in diameter. The measurements and the skin markings are checked and adjusted as necessary. The patient is re-positioned, taking great care to place the breast in exactly the same position as in the previous views. When accurate localization has been achieved, the marks on the skin are made more prominent and permanent. The 5 cm diameter images on xerographic plates will require a negative developing cycle on density 'C' to avoid excessive edge enhancement.

4 PHYSICS OF MAMMOGRAPHY

D.R. Dance and R. Davis

INTRODUCTION

Mammographic techniques have advanced rapidly during the past decade and the radiologist is faced with a choice from a wide range of equipment and methods. This chapter describes the physical characteristics of mammographic systems and it is hoped that it will aid the selection and correct use of such equipment.

In order to assess an imaging system, it is necessary to develop performance criteria and we have assumed that the visibility of calcifications (particularly, fine particles down to a size of 100 μm), and small differences in tissue density is important (Millis *et al.*, 1976). Visibility can be assessed in terms of resolution and contrast but it is also necessary to consider the perception of abnormality against a background of normal breast architecture. The approach we have adopted, therefore, is to discuss basic physical properties and to supplement this with results obtained from images of patients and of suitable breast phantoms.

Concern has been expressed about the radiation dose received by the breast during mammographic procedures. Upton *et al.* (1977) estimate that a dose of 1 rad per year starting at age 35 might increase the life-time risk of breast cancer for American women from the natural risk of 7.6% to perhaps 7.9–8.3%. It is important, therefore, that radiation dose be minimized. Unfortunately, the requirements of low dose and good image quality are in conflict and a compromise must be reached. We do not think that it is possible at present to state definitely which way this compromise should be biased and have not recommended a 'best buy' mammographic system. We have, however, suggested suitable combinations of mammographic equipment and have indicated their advantages and disadvantages.

COMPONENTS OF MAMMOGRAPHIC IMAGING SYSTEMS

The female breast is conventionally examined in cranio-caudad and medio-lateral views although other projections are often employed (see

Chapter 3). The X-ray set may be a general purpose machine or one designed for mammography, but whichever is employed, it is essential that it has an appropriate X-ray spectrum and a small focal spot. The radiation field is usually limited by a cone which may be approximately D-shaped or rectangular, and should minimize irradiation of tissue outside the field of interest. The breast should be compressed to reduce radiation dose, to enhance detail and contrast, and to reduce patient movement. This compression can be achieved by using a balloon or thin plastic sheet attached to the end of the cone or by a separate paddle device. The breast rests on a support which should have low X-ray absorption and the receptor is placed as close as possible to this support. In many cases, the cassette holding the receptor can be placed in contact with the breast, and this is to be preferred. Three types of receptor are currently in use: film, film/screen combinations and Xerox plates, and they have widely differing physical properties. After exposure, the latent image on the receptor must be developed and illuminated for viewing.

The physical characteristics of mammographic systems depend upon the combined properties of their components (Haus *et al.*, 1977). For example, unsharpness in the final image depends upon patient movement, the focal spot of the X-ray tube, the geometry used and the characteristics of the receptor. Overall contrast depends upon the composition and thickness of the object, the X-ray spectrum, scatter, detector response and image development. Each component of the complete system must be compatible with the characteristics of the other components. In this chapter we first describe the properties of the separate components and then consider complete imaging systems. Finally we discuss some of the newer developments in mammography which are still being evaluated.

Physical properties of the breast

The interaction of X-ray photons with the breast depends upon breast composition and size, and upon photon energy. In infancy the female breast is principally composed of adipose tissue but at puberty fibroglandular tissue begins to develop. This development continues until maturity but with further increase of age, the fibroglandular tissue degenerates and is gradually replaced by fat. Breast dimensions vary with population and degree of compression and at our centre the thickness of the compressed breast lies in the range 2–8 cm with a median value of about 5 cm. The breast image is approximately D-shaped and corresponds to cross-sectional areas of typically 35–270 cm² with a median value of 93 cm².

In the mammographic energy range, the principal interactions of the X-ray photons with tissue are Compton scattering and the photoelectric effect, with Compton scattering predominating at the higher energies and photoelectric absorption at the lower energies. Fig. 4.1 shows how the transmission of primary X-rays through the breast varies with thickness, composition and photon energy and was calculated using the photon

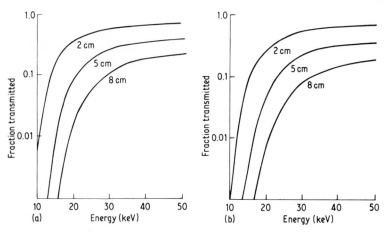

Fig. 4.1   Fraction of incident monoenergetic photons which pass through 2, 5 and 8 cm of tissue without an interaction. Curves are given for (a) adipose tissue and (b) average breast tissue which is assumed to be a 50:50 mixture by weight of adipose and fibroglandular tissue.

interaction data of Storm and Israel (1970) and the breast chemical compositions of Hammerstein *et al.* (1979). Transmission is highest for fatty tissue and lowest for fibroglandular tissue and decreases with decreasing photon energy. At energies below 15 keV very little radiation penetrates even the thinnest fatty breast. Transmission also decreases with increasing breast thickness and vigorous compression is needed to minimize radiation dose. For very thick or glandular breasts, it may be necessary to use a higher energy to improve transmission (Dance and Day, 1981).

Some of the X-ray photons which scatter in the breast can reach the detector and contribute to the image. They produce a background signal which reduces both image contrast and radiation dose. Barnes and Brezovich (1978) have measured the ratio of secondary to primary radiation in the plane of the detector for a variety of mammographic X-ray spectra. They found that it varied little with energy but increased with increasing field size to a plateau value. The contrast, or dose reductions corresponding to this plateau value were 30% and 45% for Perspex phantom thicknesses of 3 cm and 6 cm respectively. Compression therefore improves contrast by reducing scatter.

Mammographic imaging systems should have good contrast for calcifications and small tissue density differences. Fig. 4.2 shows how the contrast for a 100 μm calcification and for 1 mm of tissue vary with energy. It is clear that the requirements of low dose (Fig. 4.1) and high contrast (Fig. 4.2) are in direct conflict.

Dose specification

Radiation exposure or radiation dose to the breast can be expressed in a variety of ways and, to avoid confusion, it is important to define the

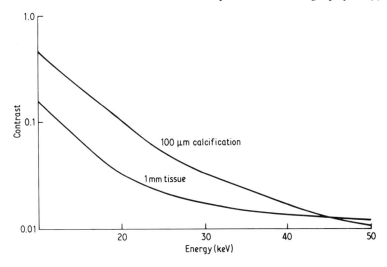

Fig. 4.2   Contrast for a 100 μm calcification (assumed to be calcium phosphate) and for 1 mm of breast tissue. The curves are for monoenergetic incident photons and contrast is taken to be (signal-background) divided by background. A correction has been applied for scattered photons corresponding to 5 cm of breast tissue.

quantity used when quoting numerical values. Equally, when assessing radiation doses, it should be checked that equivalent quantities are being compared.

The easiest quantity to measure is incident exposure which can be determined with the patient present or absent. The two values so obtained are related by the back-scatter factor (Dubuque *et al.*, 1977) which, depending on beam quality and breast size, can be as large as 1.27. Exposure is a convenient quantity but gives information about dose to air and it is better to quote radiation dose to the breast, which is related to exposure by the *f*-factor. This parameter converts from röntgens to rads and its magnitude depends upon radiation quality and tissue composition. In the mammographic energy range, variation with quality is small but variation with tissue composition is quite large. Typical values of the *f*-factor for water, fat, fibroglandular tissue and 'average breast' (assumed to be a 50:50 mixture by weight of fat and fibroglandular tissue) are 0.89, 0.52, 0.79 and 0.66 rads/R respectively (Hammerstein *et al.*, 1979). It is essential, therefore, to specify tissue type when quoting dose.

Radiation dose within the breast changes rapidly with depth and the magnitude of this variation depends upon the quality of the radiation. For example, the percentage depth doses measured at the exit from a 6 cm thick 'average breast' phantom varied between about 13% and 1% depending upon beam quality (Hammerstein *et al.*, 1979). This means that incident dose is not representative of the dose to the whole breast and should not be used to compare doses for different beam qualities. Various quantities have been suggested as being a more appropriate measure of dose: mid-breast dose, mean dose to the whole breast, mean dose to fibroglandular tissue and mean dose to the ductal parenchyma. These parameters, however, cannot be measured on a patient and use must be made of conversion tables based on phantom measurements or calculation. Such tables are only valid for simple models of the breast, but nevertheless, give a better indication of dose to the whole breast than does surface dose. Fig. 4.3 shows how the conversion factor for incident exposure to mean breast dose varies with radiation quality. The mean dose is for a breast of average composition 5 cm thick and is based on the work of Dance (1980).

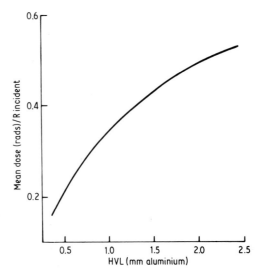

Fig. 4.3   Factor for converting incident exposure (without backscatter) to mean dose within a 5 cm thick breast. The model breast used to calculate these factors had a composition of 50% adipose and 50% fibroglandular tissue.

Mean breast dose is directly related to risk of carcinogenesis if it is assumed that all tissue is at equal risk. It is likely, however, that some tissues within the breast will be more at risk than others. Hammerstein *et al.* (1979) suggest that glandular tissue is the tissue at risk whereas Stanton *et al.* (1979) favour the ductal parenchyma. We shall ignore this complication and use mean dose to the whole breast because of the difficulty of knowing the location and composition of tissues of a particular type. The ratios of conversion factors for different models should vary little with quality (Dance, 1980) and comparisons based on mean breast dose should be similar to those based on other models.

The conventional units of exposure and dose are the röntgen and the rad and these are the units employed throughout this chapter. However, with the introduction of SI units, it may be necessary to convert from one system of units to the other. The appropriate conversion factors are: 1 röntgen = 2.58×10^{-4} coulomb kg^{-1} and 1 rad = 0.01 gray.

X-ray spectra

The mammographic energy range is approximately 15–50 keV. At the lower energy most of the radiation is absorbed in the breast and does not reach the receptor. At the higher energy contrast is reduced because of the decreasing magnitude of photoelectric absorption. Within the energy range, the shape of the spectrum may be modified by choice of anode material, filter and peak kilovoltage.

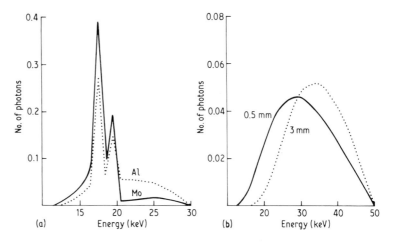

Fig. 4.4   Photon spectra for radiation from molybdenum and tungsten targets (a) molybdenum target 30 kVp with added filters of (i) 30 μm molybdenum and (ii) 0.5 mm aluminium, (b) tungsten target 50 kVp with added filters of (i) 0.5 mm aluminium and (ii) 3 mm aluminium. In each case the inherent filtration is equivalent to 0.6 mm of aluminium. The spectra are based on Fewell and Shuping (1979).

Three anode materials are currently available: molybdenum, tungsten and a molybdenum/tungsten alloy, and typical mammographic X-ray spectra have been measured by Marshal *et al.* (1975) and Fewell and Shuping (1979). Fig. 4.4 shows spectra for radiation from molybdenum and tungsten targets. The molybdenum spectrum exhibits peaks at 17.4 and 19.6 keV due to characteristic K_α and K_β X-rays and has a continuous bremsstrahlung background. The characteristic X-rays for molybdenum occur at energies where the contrast is high (Fig. 4.2) and, in general, are well suited to mammography. Molybdenum tubes usually have beryllium windows and added filters of either molybdenum or aluminium although other materials are currently being investigated. In all cases the total filtration should satisfy ICRP 15 (1970) which requires it to be equivalent to at least 0.5 mm aluminium. The effects of molybdenum and aluminium filters on the spectrum are very different (Fig. 4.4(a)). Molybdenum has a K-absorption edge at 20 keV and absorbs radiation at and above this energy very strongly and thus produces a spectrum which is dominated by the characteristic X-ray lines. Aluminium filters, however, increase the contribution of higher energy photons relative to lower energy photons. Typical filter thicknesses are 0.03 mm of molybdenum and/or 0.5–1.0 mm of aluminium. The addition of more aluminium filtration may be inappropriate because of limitations imposed by tube output and because the combined effect of filter and a thick or dense breast may mean the absorption of most of the characteristic radiation before it reaches the detector.

In quoting filter thickness, it is important to include both inherent and added filtration. It is also useful to give the measured kilovoltage and half value thickness as an indication of quality. Typical half value layers for molybdenum targets are in the range 0.30–0.90 mm Al (based on Fewell and Shuping, 1979, and the BENT manual, 1978). Half value layers should always be measured with the compression device in place as this will also filter the radiation before it reaches the breast.

The spectrum from tungsten anode tubes has peaks below 12 keV due to characteristic L X-rays and a continuous bremsstrahlung spectrum which is more intense than that from molybdenum (tungsten K X-rays occur at an energy higher than 50 keV and are not seen in mammographic spectra). It is important that the L X-rays are filtered out and do not reach the breast. The tube should therefore have a glass window; a beryllium window is unacceptable. Aluminium filters may be used to modify the spectrum (Fig. 4.4(b)) and total filtrations in the 0.5–3.0 mm range have been used depending upon the peak kilovoltage and detector employed. Half value layers for tungsten target tubes typically lie in the range 0.38–3.0 mm aluminium (based on the BENT manual, 1978, and Fitzgerald et al., 1979).

The molybdenum/tungsten alloy target has properties intermediate between those of its components. However, we are not aware of any published evaluation of the performance of this alloy target and in the following sections have avoided commenting on its suitability. In all cases contrast and dose would be intermediate between those produced by its separate components under the same conditions.

The choice of spectrum will depend upon contrast and radiation dose: Table 4.1 gives contrast calculated for a 100 μm calcification and Fig. 4.5 shows how the dose within the breast varies with depth, tissue type and radiation quality. Once again, these data indicate that the requirements of high contrast and low dose are in conflict. As the radiation becomes harder, the transmission of radiation through the breast increases and dose decreases, but contrast decreases as well. For very thick glandular breasts, the softest radiation can be heavily absorbed and will then contribute little to contrast but a lot to dose.

In conclusion, radiation from a molybdenum target can give the best

Table 4.1   Contrast for 100 μm calcification. Results are given for three
thicknesses of average breast tissue and four radiation qualities. The contrast
was calculated as for Fig. 4.2 and corresponds to the number of photons
leaving the breast.

kVp	Target	Added filtration	HVL mm Al	Contrast for 100 μm calcification		
				2 cm breast	5 cm breast	8 cm breast
30	Mo	0.03 mm Mo	0.36	0.15	0.090	0.050
45	Mo	0.03 mm Mo	0.52	0.083	0.038	0.020
35	W	—	0.90	0.070	0.046	0.030
50	W	2.0 mm Al	2.07	0.033	0.023	0.015

contrast and radiation from a tungsten target the least dose. The final
choice of spectrum, however, will also depend upon the contrast
enhancement properties and sensitivity of the receptor employed.

Direct exposure film receptors

At the present time film/screen or Xerox receptors are used in the majority
of mammographic examinations in Britain (Fitzgerald *et al.*, 1979) and in
the USA (Jans *et al.*, 1979). The use of film receptors without a screen is
small because of the high dose associated with the technique and our
treatment here is correspondingly brief.

The properties of mammographic films are discussed in the BENT
manual (1978) and by Gajewski (1977).

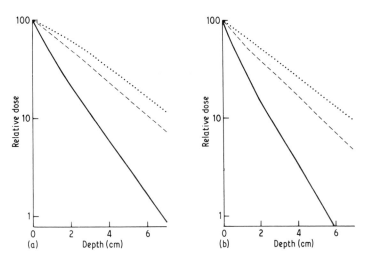

Fig. 4.5   Variation of breast dose with depth and radiation quality for (a)
adipose tissue and (b) 'average breast' tissue. The upper curves are for a
tungsten target at 50 kVp (HVL 1.21 mm aluminium). The middle curves are
for a tungsten target at 40 kVp (HVL 0.79 mm aluminium). The lower curves
are for a molybdenum target at 28 kVp (HVL 0.31 mm of aluminium). The
curves are based on the work of Hammerstein *et al.* (1979).

Resolution and contrast

Direct exposure films for mammography should exhibit good resolution
and high contrast. They should therefore be fine grained with little
variation in grain size and should have a thick double emulsion to
minimize radiation dose. These criteria are satisfied by certain industrial
X-ray films and by films specially designed for mammography. Using
such films, the resolution of the overall imaging system is limited by the
size of the X-ray tube focal spot.

The contrast enhancement of photographic film is usually expressed in
terms of the slope of the characteristic curve. Fig. 4.6(a) shows a typical
curve for a direct exposure mammographic film. Its important features are
its steep gradient which increases with density and its narrow latitude.

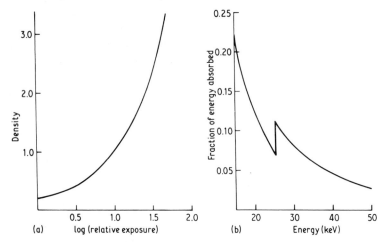

Fig. 4.6   Properties of direct exposure mammographic films. (a) Typical
characteristic curve. (b) Fraction of incident energy which is absorbed in an
emulsion thickness of 5 mg cm^{-2} of silver bromide.

Maximum contrast enhancement can be obtained by using the steepest
portion of the curve and exposing films to a greater density than normal
(up to 3.0 D). The films produced using this high density technique must
be viewed using a high intensity illuminator. Gajewski (1977) recom-
mends that the maximum available viewing intensity be not less than
6000 cd m^{-2} and points out that it is important to use masking to reduce
glare. If a mammographic film is exposed to a low density, the contrast is
reduced and the visibility of small detail in the image will be impaired.

The narrow latitude of the films is a limitation because the compressed
breast has regions of very different density. Correct exposure is therefore
important and this can most easily be achieved by the use of automatic
exposure termination. An alternative approach is the use of a 'dual-pack'
containing films of two different speeds. These are exposed together and
provide information about breast regions of high and low density.

Sensitivity

The sensitivity of an X-ray film is determined by its grain size, packing density, emulsion thickness, X-ray absorption efficiency and development. The fine grain size of direct exposure mammographic films means that they are slow and a high X-ray absorption coefficient is therefore important.

The principal interaction between photons in the mammographic energy range and silver bromide is the photoelectric effect. This can be accompanied by the emission of photoelectrons, Auger electrons or fluorescent X-ray photons from the silver or bromine atoms. If these particles deposit energy within a grain they contribute to the image, but otherwise their energy is wasted. Fortunately, electron ranges are short but fluorescent photons can travel further and some can escape the emulsion layer and do not contribute to the image. Fig. 4.6(b) shows the calculated energy absorption coefficient for an emulsion thickness of $5\ mg\ cm^{-2}$, due allowance having been made for the absorption or escape of fluorescent X-ray photons (Dance, unpublished). The discontinuity in the curve occurs at the K-absorption edge for silver which is the threshold energy for X-ray photons to eject an electron from the innermost shell of the silver atom. At this point 40% of the energy of the interacting photons is lost to escaping fluorescent photons. The figure shows that the energy absorption coefficient of film is low and is not well matched to the spectra from X-ray tubes with tungsten or molybdenum targets.

Film/screen receptors

Mammographic film/screen combinations are faster than direct exposure films but do not have such a good inherent resolution. Nevertheless, if an appropriate screen is used in the correct configuration, good quality films may be obtained.

The properties of film/screen systems are outlined in the BENT manual (1978) and by Webster and Kalisher (1977).

Resolution and contrast

Most of the blackening of a film exposed in contact with a screen is due to the fluorescent light photons emitted by the screen and it is these photons which limit the resolution of the technique. Direct interactions with the film emulsion contribute only a few per cent of the total blackening. Following interactions in the screen, the fluorescent photons produced are emitted isotropically and spread out as they travel from screen to emulsion, their spread being proportional to the distance between the point of production and the film. This distance should therefore be reduced as much as possible and this can be achieved as follows:

(a) A single screen is used with a single emulsion film. This configuration eliminates the crossover effect associated with double screen/double emulsion techniques.

(b) Good contact is maintained between the screen and the emulsion (Weiss and Wayrynen, 1976).

(c) The screen is placed behind the film. More X-ray photons interact in the front half of the screen than in the back half and this configuration brings the production point of the fluorescent light photons as close as possible to the emulsion.

(d) The screen construction is optimized. The spread of fluorescent photons depends upon the thickness of the fluorescent layer and the presence or absence of any reflecting layers or absorptive dyes. These parameters are selected by the manufacturer and influence resolution and sensitivity. To obtain adequate resolution it is essential that a film/screen combination specifically recommended for mammography be used.

The contrast associated with film/screen combinations is high although the shape of the characteristic curve (Fig. 4.7(a)) is different from that of a directly exposed film. Because the exposure is made by light photons, the gradient of the curve, or film gamma, has a maximum at an intermediate density and then decreases in magnitude. As a consequence, the high density technique suggested for direct exposure films is inappropriate.

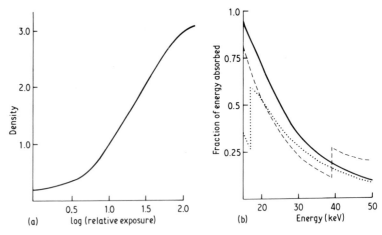

Fig. 4.7   Properties of mammographic film/screen combinations. (a) Typical characteristic curve. (b) Fraction of incident energy which is absorbed in a screen 100 μm thick with a 50% packing density. Curves are given for calcium tungstate and gadolinium oxysulphide (———), lanthanum oxysulphide (------), and yttrium oxysulphide (·······). The curves for calcium tungstate and gadolinium oxysulphide are so similar that they have been superimposed.

The gammas of film/screen combinations may not be as high as those of direct exposure films and their latitude not quite as narrow (BENT manual, 1978) but it is still important to obtain the correct exposure if breast regions of both high and low density are to be properly imaged.

Sensitivity of the screen

Modern mammographic screens have a fluorescent layer of either calcium tungstate (e.g. Du Pont Lo-dose, Ostrum *et al.*, 1973) or a terbium activated rare-earth phosphor (e.g. Kodak Min-R, Chang *et al.*, 1976).

Their sensitivity is determined by their X-ray absorption characteristics and light production efficiency. Fig. 4.7(b) shows calculated energy absorption coefficients for screens 100 μm thick with a 50% phosphor packing density. Curves are given for calcium tungstate and for gadolinium, lanthanum and yttrium oxysulphides. In the mammographic energy range, X-ray photons primarily undergo photoelectric interactions with the screen phosphor and the coefficients were calculated as described earlier for direct exposure film. Calcium tungstate and gadolinium oxysulphide have the best energy absorption efficiencies and their curves show no discontinuities. The efficiency of yttrium oxysulphide is lower and shows a discontinuity at the yttrium K-absorption edge at 17.0 keV which is the threshold for the ejection of photoelectrons from the K-shell. There is an increase in photoelectric absorption at this energy but some of the energy from the interacting photons is carried off by K-fluorescent X-ray photons. (These should not be confused with the fluorescent light photons which expose the film emulsion). In fact, at the K-edge, 30% of the energy of the interacting photon escapes the screen. This percentage decreases with energy and is 10% at 50 keV. Those K-fluorescent photons which are absorbed in the screen will in general travel some distance from their production point before being absorbed. This means that for the same screen thickness, the line spread response function for the yttrium phosphor will have broader wings than that for the gadolinium phosphor. Similar comments can be made for lanthanum oxysulphide, but in this case the K-edge is at a higher energy.

The overall sensitivity of a screen also depends on the efficiency with which the energy absorbed is converted to light. This efficiency will depend upon screen thickness and the presence or absence of absorptive dyes and reflecting layers but for an idealized screen is 3.5% for calcium tungstate and 15%, 12% and 18% for gadolinium, lanthanum and yttrium oxysulphides respectively (Stevels, 1975). It will be seen that the overall sensitivity difference between rare-earth and tungstate screens 100 μm thick can be a factor of 3–5. Comparing the various rare-earth phosphors, gadolinium and yttrium oxysulphide should have the best overall efficiency but the resolution of the gadolinium salt should be superior. The increased sensitivity of the rare-earth phosphors can in principle be utilized to reduce dose or improve resolution but, in practice, the advantage achieved is small. This is because mammographic film/screen systems are noise limited and sensitivity has to be sacrificed in order to reduce quantum mottle.

Sensitivity of the film

The wavelength spectrum of the fluorescent light photons emitted by a screen depends upon the phosphor material used. The spectra given by Stevels (1975) show that the light emitted by gadolinium and lanthanum oxysulphides is predominantly green whereas light from calcium tungstate is blue. The spectrum from yttrium oxysulphide is mainly green but can be shifted towards the blue at low concentrations of the terbium activator.

For maximum sensitivity the spectral response of the film should be matched to the light emitted by the screen. The films conventionally used with radiographic screens are predominantly blue sensitive and are not suitable for use with screens emitting green light. An orthochromatic film should be used in such cases. In practice, however, maximum sensitivity may not be required and the film may be used to control the overall efficiency.

Quantum mottle

If a film/screen system is exposed to a uniform X-ray beam, the image produced will show small variations in density. The principle source of these fluctuations is the statistical variation in the number of X-ray photons absorbed per unit area of the screen and the effect is known as quantum mottle because of its radiographic appearance. This feature has been investigated for rare-earth screens by Wagner and Weaver (1976). The magnitude of the mottle depends upon the number of photons interacting per unit area of the screen and upon its frequency response. As the number of interacting photons decreases and as the frequency response increases so the mottle increases.

The most important consequence of quantum mottle in mammography is decreased visibility of small objects. In fact the noise level in film/screen mammographic images can be comparable in magnitude to the signal from a small calcification (Moores, 1980). The design of a screen is therefore a balance between sensitivity, noise and resolution, and it may not be possible to fully utilize the high light output of rare-earth phosphors. For noise-limited imaging a high energy absorption coefficient (Fig. 4.7(b)) is more important than a high screen sensitivity.

Practical considerations

To achieve good resolution, it is essential to ensure contact between screen and emulsion. This is normally achieved by vacuum packaging in light tight plastic bags but cassettes are also available which bring the screen in contact with the emulsion. X-ray absorption in the vacuum packing and in the cassettes is similar. For both methods cleanliness is important as dust particles can produce artefacts on the film (although with experience, these can normally be distinguished from calcification).

Screen films are suitable for automatic development but in the case of green sensitive emulsions it is important to use a special safelight.

Xeroradiography

Xeroradiography is a dry non-silver photographic process which can enhance fine detail and small differences in contrast and yet has a wide exposure latitude. It is well suited to mammography where calcifications and small tissue density differences need to be visualized against a background of variable tissue thickness.

The physical principles of the technique have been reviewed by Boag (1973(a) and 1975) and Seelentag (1979) and its application in mammography discussed by Wolfe (1972). The use of the commercially available Xerox 125 System is described in the manufacturer's technical bulletins (Xerox Corporation, 1974 onwards).

Formation of the latent image

The image receptor supplied by the Xerox Corporation is a sheet of amorphous selenium 135 μm thick deposited uniformly on an aluminium backing plate. The surface of the selenium is given a uniform positive electric charge and the plate is then enclosed in a light tight cassette. Because selenium is a photoconductor, the charge will then remain on the surface of the plate until it is irradiated. (In practice there is a small dark current and the surface charge will slowly leak through the selenium with a half discharge time in excess of one hour). When the plate is exposed to X-rays, the energy absorbed from the incident photons liberates electrons and holes within the bulk of the material. These charge carriers migrate towards the surface of the plate under the influence of the electric field within the selenium and thus a photon-induced electric current flows (photoconductivity). This current causes a discharge of the plate so that a latent image of the pattern of the incident photons is formed by subtraction from the original uniform charge distribution.

Sensitivity

Selenium is a suitable photoconducting material for xeroradiography because it can be deposited uniformly and in sufficient thickness on the backing plate to achieve a high photon absorption efficiency. Most of the interactions of the incident X-ray photons with the selenium atoms are photoelectric and may be accompanied by the emission of K-fluorescent X-ray photons, some of which can escape from the plate. Our calculations indicate that at 15 keV 10% of the energy of an interacting photon is lost in this way. Fig. 4.8 shows the fraction of the energy incident on the selenium which is absorbed and the equivalent result for a calcium tungstate screen 100 μm thick. The energy absorption efficiency of the selenium plate is

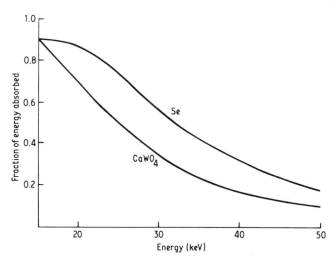

Fig. 4.8   Fraction of the incident energy which is absorbed in the Xerox plate. Also shown is the same fraction for a calcium tungstate screen 100 μm thick with a 50% packing density.

superior and this is largely because of the greater density and thickness of the selenium. Since, however, contrast falls with increasing photon energy, this improved sensitivity does mean a decreased inherent contrast in the latent image when compared with that of a film or film/screen combination irradiated with the same photon pattern.

The efficiency for conversion of energy absorbed in the Xerox plate to neutralized surface charge, depends upon the strength of the electric field in the selenium; the stronger the field, the greater the efficiency (Fender, 1975). This means that it is important to give the plate a high surface charge before irradiation. As the selenium is irradiated and discharges so the charge neutralized per unit energy decreases and the overall efficiency falls. This property contributes to the wide latitude of the technique.

Powder development

The latent or charge image on the selenium plate is developed with an aerosol of fine particles of a blue powder. These toner particles are charged by friction and are attracted by the charge distributed on the surface of the receptor. In this way a powder pattern is built up which is representative of the latent image. The development process is controlled by a back bias voltage which is applied to the rear of the plate and can add to or subtract from the latent image and thus produces either positive or negative radiographs (for examples, see Chapter 6). In the positive image mode, the more highly charged areas correspond to the dense parts of the object and are dark blue, whereas, the discharged areas, which correspond to the less dense parts of the object, are light blue. In the negative mode, the opposite configuration is obtained.

Image characteristics

Powder developed xeroradiographs show low contrast between large areas of different density because the whole plate is exposed to a powder cloud but show marked enhancement in the vicinity of any sharp change in contrast. This phenomenon is known as edge enhancement and may be understood by reference to Fig. 4.9 which shows the lines of electric force in the region of a step in the electric charge. To a good approximation the charged toner particles follow the lines of force and so will be heaped on one side of the charge step and deficient on the other. The image will therefore be dark blue on one side of a step and white on the other. Edge enhancement is of great value in mammography since it facilitates the perception of calcifications and of edges between tissues of different density.

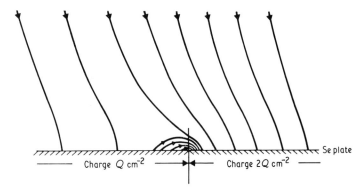

Fig. 4.9   Enlarged view of lines of electric force in the vicinity of a charge step on the surface of a selenium plate. Based on Boag (1973b). There is a grounded electrode (not shown in the figure) which is distant from the selenium plate. (Reproduced with permission from Butterworth and Co (Publishers) Ltd.)

The degree of edge enhancement is usually expressed in terms of the width of the white band or halo at a density step. This depends upon the initial voltage on the plate, the exposure itself and the back bias voltage applied during development (Zeman *et al.*, 1976). It is important that these be optimized to obtain the best performance from the system. Whilst the technique has a wide latitude, allowing both skin and chest wall to be well visualized on the same image, the visibility of fine detail will depend upon exposure (Ramsden *et al.*, 1979). For images of the highest quality, as much care in exposure is required as for a conventional radiograph. A useful rule of thumb for the positive mode is that the properly exposed xerogram should have a 1 mm wide edge enhancement halo at the skin.

The Xerox plate requires a greater exposure than a mammographic film/screen system and yet has a higher photon absorption efficiency. More absorbed photons are needed to produce an acceptable image and the effect of quantum mottle should be less than in film/screen mammography.

The Xerox 125 System

The Xerox 125 System for xeroradiography consists of a conditioner and a processor. The conditioner prepares the plate for exposure by heating to remove any residual electric charge, by charging its surface and by placing it in a light tight cassette. The front face of this cassette is a carbon fibre composite designed to minimise X-ray absorption and yet to be sufficiently strong to prevent the formation of pressure artefacts in the image (De Werd, 1979). After exposure, the cassette is placed in the processor and the plate is automatically moved to a powder cloud development chamber. The powder image is transferred onto a sheet of paper by contact with the plate and is fixed permanently by heating which fuses the powder into the thermoplastic coating of the paper. The selenium plate is then cleaned ready for re-use. It should be noted that because of the contact transfer between plate and paper, the final radiograph is a mirror image.

The 125 System can be used in daylight and produces an image in 90 seconds. The radiograph is viewed in reflected light and a good level of surface illumination is essential.

A limitation of the Xerox System is the production of artefacts (De Werd, 1979). These can sometimes simulate calcifications but in most cases can be correctly identified and we have found that with good quality control, artefact production is not a serious problem.

Geometric considerations

The finite size of the X-ray tube focal spot causes a blurring of the radiographic image. This is called geometric unsharpness and its magnitude is proportional to the distance of the point of interest in the breast from the detector and to the size of the focal spot and it is important that these be minimized. The former can be reduced by compressing the breast and by placing the detector as close as possible to it. The size of the focal spot is limited by tube output requirements but should have a measured value of not more than 1 mm.

Geometric unsharpness is inversely proportional to the distance of the point of interest from the focal spot and the focus skin distance (FSD) should therefore be as large as practicable. Fig. 4.10(a) shows the modulation transfer function (MTF) for a Senographe X-ray set (focal spot size approximately 1 mm) at an FSD of 28 cm and an object receptor distance of 5 cm (Haus, 1977). Also shown are the MTFs for commercial film and film/screen receptors. The frequency response of the film is better than that of the film/screen combination, but for both detectors the overall resolution is limited by the geometry employed. Little advantage in resolution will be gained by using a film. If, however, the FSD is increased, the MTF of the X-ray set will improve. Fig. 4.10(b) shows the MTFs at an FSD of 61 cm. The overall MTF is better for both systems (in practice, direct exposure films have a low sensitivity and the FSD may

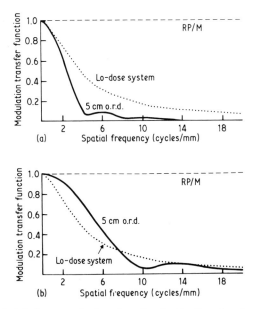

Fig. 4.10   Modulation transfer functions for the Du Pont Lo-dose film/screen system, Kodak RP/M film and geometric unsharpness. The latter curves are for an object to receptor distance (o.r.d.) of 5 cm and focus skin distances of (a) 28 cm and (b) 61 cm. Based on Haus (1977) (with permission of John Wiley and Sons, Inc.).

then be limited because of restrictions imposed by tube output and motion unsharpness).

Xeroradiography is also affected by geometric unsharpness. Boag (1975) claims that its inherent resolution is better than 50 line pairs mm^{-1} and the overall resolution is therefore limited by geometric considerations. Once again the largest possible FSD should be used, consistent with the output of the X-ray tube (Haus, 1977). We routinely use an FSD of 75 cm with our tungsten anode set (focal spot size 1 mm).

PERFORMANCE OF FILM AND FILM/SCREEN MAMMOGRAPHIC SYSTEMS

Influence of X-ray spectrum

The properties of radiation from tungsten and molybdenum targets have been discussed above where it is pointed out that contrast is better with radiation from molybdenum targets and decreases with increasing peak voltage. Radiation dose, however, decreases as the beam hardens and is least for a tungsten X-ray tube with a high peak kilovoltage. In practice, peak voltages in the range 26–35 kV can be regarded as being suitable for film and film/screen mammography (e.g. BENT manual, 1978), the higher voltages being used for the denser breasts.

Most work comparing tungsten and molybdenum is based on film receptors but the similarity of film and film/screen images allows the same conclusions to be drawn for both types of receptor. Radiographic contrast has been measured by several authors using film and molybdenum and tungsten X-ray tubes. Rini *et al.* (1973) and Evans *et al.* (1975) found superior contrast using molybdenum X-ray tubes. Haus *et al.* (1976) radiographed a specimen with scatter material added. They found that molybdenum gave better contrast than tungsten for total thicknesses of 1.5–5 cm but that the tungsten and molybdenum images had equal contrast for 8 cm of breast equivalent material. This is because most of the characteristic molybdenum radiation is absorbed in such a thickness and contributes to the radiation dose but not to the image. The images produced by the molybdenum anode tube through the 8 cm thick phantom required an exposure 20 times larger than that for the 1.5 cm thick phantom. The corresponding exposure ratio for the tungsten tube was 6.

Studies of the visibility of real (Millis *et al.*, 1976) or simulated (Evans *et al.*, 1975) calcifications show that images obtained with a molybdenum target are superior to those obtained with a tungsten target. The recent survey of Fitzgerald *et al.* (1979) confirms this: images of a breast phantom containing a variety of simulated pathology were consistently better for molybdenum anodes than for tungsten anodes. The surface dose, however, was higher for the radiation from the molybdenum target.

Commercial film and film/screen receptors

The performance of film and film/screen receptors may be evaluated in terms of their physical parameters or by imaging phantoms, specimens or patients. Moores *et al.* (1979) and Tonge *et al.* (1976) have investigated the visibility of simulated and real calcifications respectively for film and film/screen combinations. They found that visibility of small calcifications decreased as receptor sensitivity increased. The best visibility was obtained with direct exposure film, but with an associated dose penalty. On the other hand the fastest film/screen combinations had the poorest resolution and were noisy. Table 4.2 which is adapted from the work of Moores *et al.* (1979), illustrates this by showing how the detectability of simulated calcifications in a simple phantom varies with radiation dose. Table 4.3 gives measured patient exposures for several film/screen combinations, for xeroradiography and for direct exposure film.

Comparative evaluations of various film/screen combinations have also been made by Arnold *et al.* (1978) and Sickles and Genant (1979). The latter authors compared the performance of five film/screen combinations using multiple patient exposures and evaluated their results in terms of breast architecture and masses and calcifications seen. They found that the slowest system investigated, Du Pont Lo-dose I, was the best, but the differences between the five systems were small and they suggest that any of them would be suitable for mammography.

Table 4.2 Relative radiation dose and calcification detectability for various film/screen and film receptors. The particle sizes were deduced by Moores *et al.* (1979) from receiver operating characteristics (ROC curves) and correspond to a 50% true positive detection rate and a 2% false positive detection rate. Rare-earth and tungstate screens are labelled RE and T respectively.

Screen	Film	Relative dose	Particle size (μm) for 50% detection
Trimax α 4 (RE)	Trimax XD		
Agfa-Gevaert MR50 (RE)	Agfa-Gevaert Mammoray RP3	4.5	308
Ilford High Definition (T)	Agfa-Gevaert Medichrome	4.9	300
Kodak Min–R (RE)	Kodak MR–1	5.4	260
Du Pont Lo-Dose (T)	Du Pont Lo-dose	6.5	280
Trimax αM (RE)	Trimax XM	17.5	248
	Kodak Industrex C	22.7	230

It is interesting to note that the work of Arnold *et al.* (1978) and Moores *et al.* (1979) suggests that the resolution of rare earth film/screen systems is slightly better than that of tungstate film/screen systems of similar efficiency.

Conclusions for film and film/screen combinations

(a) The FSD should be as long as practicable.

(b) Radiographs taken with radiation from a molybdenum anode tube show superior contrast to those taken with a tungsten anode tube. The difference in contrast decreases with increasing breast thickness and is small for radiologically dense breasts. Unfortunately, breast dose is higher for mammography using a molybdenum tube and this dose disadvantage increases with breast thickness. Nevertheless, we recommend that if just one X-ray tube is to be used for film or film/screen mammography, molybdenum is the most appropriate anode material.

(c) The radiation dose for examinations made with film/screen systems is 5–20 times less than that for direct exposure film systems. This considerable advantage is only partly offset by the superior resolution and noise properties of direct exposure films.

PERFORMANCE OF XEROMAMMOGRAPHIC SYSTEMS

Influence of X-ray spectrum

The choice of the most appropriate X-ray spectrum for xeromammography is not simple. Because edge enhancement improves the

Table 4.3 Breast exposure and dose corresponding to various receptors and radiation qualities. The exposures include backscatter and are averages over a series of patients for a single cranio-caudad view. The film/screen exposures are taken from Sickles and Genant (1979) and the remaining exposures are taken from work at our own centre. The mean doses correspond to a 5 cm thick breast of 'average' composition and the conversion factors were deduced from Dance (1980).

Image receptor	Radiation quality				Surface exposure (R)	Mean dose (rads)
	Target	kVp	Added filtration	HVL, mm Al		
Screen/film						
Du Pont Lo-dose/Lo-dose	Mo	35	0.03 mm Mo		1.3	0.21
Du Pont Lo-dose II/Lo dose	Mo	35	0.03 mm Mo		0.64	0.11
Kodak Min-R/MR-1	Mo	35	0.03 mm Mo		0.57	0.09
Xerox						
Xerox positive mode	Mo	45	0.03 mm Mo	0.52	6.7	1.3
Xerox positive mode	Mo	45	0.03 mm Mo + 0.9 mm Al	0.67	3.0	0.7
Xerox positive mode	W	45	0	1.11	1.5	0.49
Xerox positive mode	W	45	1.8 mm Al	1.78	1.0	0.42
Xerox negative mode	W	45	0	1.11	1.1	0.36
Film						
Kodak PE4006	Mo	30	0.03 mm Mo		12	1.9

perception of small details and because the efficiency of a Xerox plate does not fall off as rapidly with energy as the efficiency of a mammographic screen (Fig. 4.8), it is possible to use radiation which is harder than that used for film and film/screen mammography. As the radiation hardens, the dose to the breast decreases but image contrast becomes less marked and the choice of quality is a compromise between these two effects. The usual tube potential employed in xeromammography lies in the range 35–50 kVp for both molybdenum and tungsten targets. The Xerox Corporation suggest that 2–3 mm of aluminium filtration be added to tubes with tungsten targets to further harden the radiation: the associated reduction in edge enhancement being largely compensated by changing the back bias voltage which controls development (Xerox Corporation Technical Application Bulletin No. 5, 1976). The addition of a similar thickness of aluminium filtration to a tube with a molybdenum target would modify the radiation spectrum so much that for medium to thick breasts very little of the molybdenum characteristic radiation would reach the detector. Table 4.3 shows how breast exposure and dose depend upon radiation quality. It is clear that a considerable dose advantage can be achieved using a tungsten target with additional filtration.

The effect of beam hardness on the quality of the xeromammogram has been investigated in various ways, none of which encompass all the factors which need to be considered. Evans *et al.* (1975) have compared mammograms of patients taken with tungsten and molybdenum tubes at 35 kVp and found the two sets of images to be of equal quality. Tonge *et al.* (1976), Ramsden *et al.* (1979) and Stanton *et al.* (1979) have investigated the visibility of real or simulated calcifications. Their results show that the threshold size for visibility increases as the radiation quality hardens but lies in the range of 100–200 μm for radiation from both molybdenum and tungsten targets. (This size range should not be compared directly with the data in Table 4.2 which use a different measure of visibility.) The above investigations were made without compensating for loss of contrast by adjusting the back bias voltage. The Xerox Corporation found that the addition of 2–3 mm of aluminium filtration to a beam from a tungsten target together with a change in back bias voltage made only a small difference to calcification visibility (Xerox Corporation Technical Application Bulletin No. 5, 1976). This result has been confirmed by studies on patients by van de Riet and Wolfe (1977) and by ourselves (Davis *et al.* 1980), which indicate that although the appearance of the mammogram is altered, its diagnostic efficacy is unimpaired.

Choice of development mode

Xeroradiography is a non-linear process and images developed in the positive and negative modes are not complementary. The principal difference between the two modes is their edge enhancement (Xerox Corporation Technical Application Bulletin No. 7, 1977). For positive images, the white halo associated with an edge occurs in the region which corresponds to the lesser tissue density. For negative images it occurs in the region with the greater tissue density. If there are large density differences within the breast, the edge enhancement halo can be quite wide and can obscure detail in the image. For example, small calcifications imaged in the negative mode can have their internal structure masked by the edge enhancement halo and this can make it difficult to distinguish calcification from artefact.

The radiation dose associated with negative mode imaging is 20–30% less than that for the positive mode (Table 4.3 and Buchanan and Jager, 1977).

Conclusions for xeromammography

(a) The FSD should be as long as practicable.

(b) Good quality mammograms can be obtained using radiation from either molybdenum or tungsten tubes. However, the mean breast dose associated with the use of a molybdenum anode is greater than that for a tungsten anode. We recommend that a tungsten anode be used and that a total filtration of approximately 2 mm of aluminium be used.

(c) Negative mode mammograms require less dose than those developed in the positive mode but a detailed clinical comparison of the two modes has not yet appeared in the literature.

RECENT DEVELOPMENTS

Magnification techniques

When using conventional X-ray tubes it is important to place the detector as close as possible to the breast to minimize geometric unsharpness. However, this rule can be relaxed if an ultra fine focus tube is used. For example, the tube manufactured by RSI, which has a tungsten target and a measured focal spot size of 220 μm × 190 μm, has been used by Sickles *et al.* (1977) to give a magnification of 1.5.

Geometric unsharpness increases with increasing magnification, but can remain comparable to detector unsharpness if the focal spot is small enough. Since the image of breast detail is enlarged, the effective resolution of the magnification technique can then be superior to that obtained with conventional geometry. For the same reason, the effect of quantum noise on the image is also reduced. As the gap between breast and detector increases, so the contribution of scatter to the image decreases and the contrast improves. Sickles *et al.* (1977) found that this improvement was small for a magnification of 1.5 but Arnold *et al.* (1979) claim that at a magnification of 2.0, the increased gap removed 75% of the scatter.

On the debit side, the output of fine focus tubes is low and long exposures may be necessary. Radiation dose is increased because the image is spread over a greater area of the detector and contrast will be reduced if a tungsten target is used with a film/screen combination. Furthermore, because the image is magnified, it may not be possible to include the whole of the breast image on one film.

Sickles *et al.* (1979) have made a detailed comparison of the magnification technique with conventional film/screen mammography using both phantom and patient studies. They claim much better visibility for both fine detail and breast architecture and have used the technique with success for breasts classified as equivocal on a conventional mammogram.

Grid techniques

Mammography is conventionally performed without a grid for the following reasons (Gajewski, 1977):

(a) The use of a grid would increase the dose to the breast.
(b) It may be more difficult to image regions close to the chest wall.
(c) Conventional grids would harden and attenuate the primary radiation too much.
(d) Geometric unsharpness would be greater because of increased separation between breast and detector.

Recently, Friedrich and Weskamp (1978) have described a new grid designed specifically for mammography which overcomes some of these objections. The grid is used with an extended FSD and a rare-earth film/screen combination. It is claimed that worthwhile improvements in contrast can be obtained for thick breasts where there is a large scatter component in the image.

Ionography

Conventional mammographic systems use a solid detector in order to achieve a high X-ray absorption efficiency but good efficiencies can be obtained using certain gaseous absorbers. This is achieved by using a gas-filled chamber with a pressure–thickness product of 5–10 atm cm. The ions produced within the gas by the incident X-rays are attracted to the surface plates of the chamber by an electric field and build up a charge pattern on an insulating foil. This process is known as ionography or electron radiography and has been reviewed by Boag (1975) and Seelentag (1979). The charge pattern can be developed using a powder cloud (Moores *et al.*, 1980) but the commercial Xonics equipment uses a liquid toner and produces images without marked edge enhancement. The breast doses quoted for the Xonics system are less than those obtained using xeroradiography or film/screen combinations (Stanton *et al.*, 1979) and this is because a sensitive charge development process is used. However, the visibilities of simulated calcifications and spicules are not as good as those obtained with xeroradiography but are claimed to be similar to those for a film/screen combination. Because of the increased sensitivity of the Xonics system, the effect of quantum noise on the image may be important, and further evaluation is required.

SUMMARY

Good quality mammography can be achieved at a low dose with either a film/screen combination and a molybdenum target or a Xerox plate and a tungsten target with extra filtration. The mean breast dose associated with mammographic film/screen combinations can be less than that associated with the Xerox technique, but the imaging characteristics of the two methods are different and the choice between them is not straightforward. Whichever system is used the breast should be compressed, the focal spot of the X-ray tube should be small and the focus skin distance should be as long as practicable.

ACKNOWLEDGEMENTS

It is a pleasure to thank Michael Fitzgerald for his detailed and constructive criticism of the text and the Medical Art Department of the Royal Marsden Hospital for preparing the diagrams.

5 MAMMOGRAPHIC FEATURES OF BENIGN DISEASE

C.A. Parsons

As much care, and possibly more care, is needed in making a benign diagnosis from a mammogram as in deciding that a lesion is malignant. The clinician reassured by the radiologist's report of benignicity may decide on a lengthy interval before reviewing the patient, or, even discharge her from his clinic. So that a false negative report could lead to an important delay in diagnosis. On the other hand, there are many radiological features of benign breast disease which are absolutely identical with the signs of malignancy, so that occasional false positive reports or, at least, reports indicating the suspicious nature of the radiological findings are inevitable.

There is remarkable aetiological variety in benign breast disease, and this is reflected in the range of mammographic features of abnormality. By far the most common condition is benign mammary dysplasia.

BENIGN MAMMARY DYSPLASIA

The study of benign mammary dysplasia (BMD) is not made easier by the nomenclature. There are at least ten synonyms for the condition, few of which are of anything but historical interest. Pathologists find cystic hyperplasia the most useful term but it does not indicate all the abnormalities seen by the radiologist. Benign mammary dysplasia embraces a number of benign physiological and pathological changes involving both epithelial and stromal elements which vary in degree clinically and radiologically throughout the menstrual cycle.

The most common radiological abnormality is increased density (Figs 5.1–5.6). This may take the form of either multiple ill-defined opacities which when surrounded by fat appear discrete, or a more homogeneous diffuse increase in density. The nodular changes may be so gross that the lesions virtually become confluent. These represent areas of adenosis with perilobular and periductal fibrosis. The changes are nearly always symmetrical. Indeed, the most common cause of lack of symmetry is previous biopsy. The condition may be difficult to recognize in the young

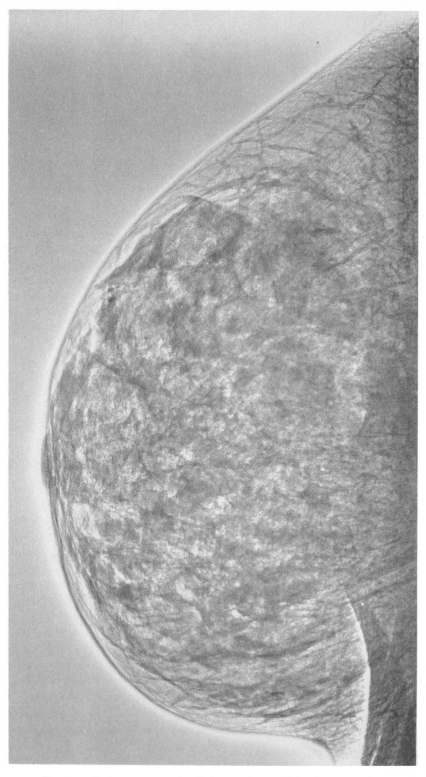

Fig. 5.1 Benign mammary dysplasia: very dense nodular tissue occupies virtually the whole of the breast. Age 36.

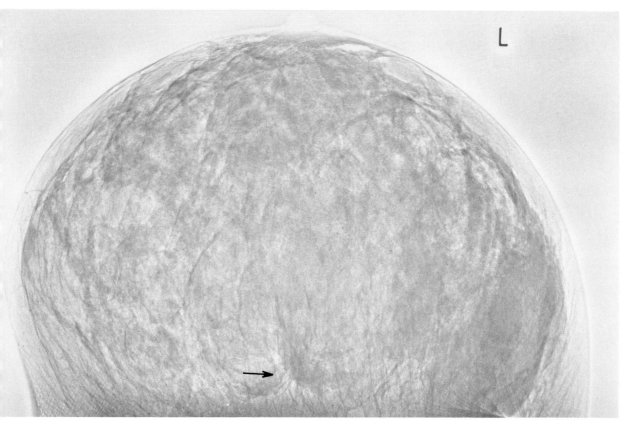

Fig. 5.2 Benign mammary dysplasia: the breast tissue is diffusely dense with a small number of centrally scattered calcifications. The spiculated area deep in the breast (arrow) represents sclerosing adenosis. Age 47.

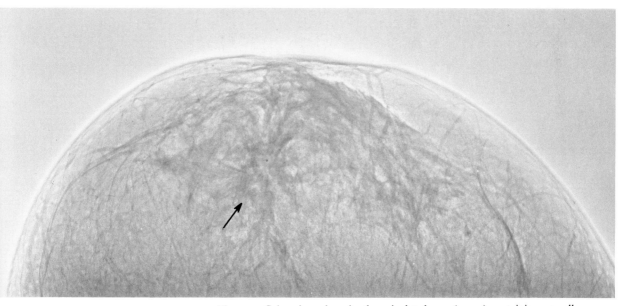

Fig. 5.3 Sclerosing adenosis: the spiculated area (arrow) containing a small number of calcifications deep to the nipple represents sclerosing adenosis. Age 52.

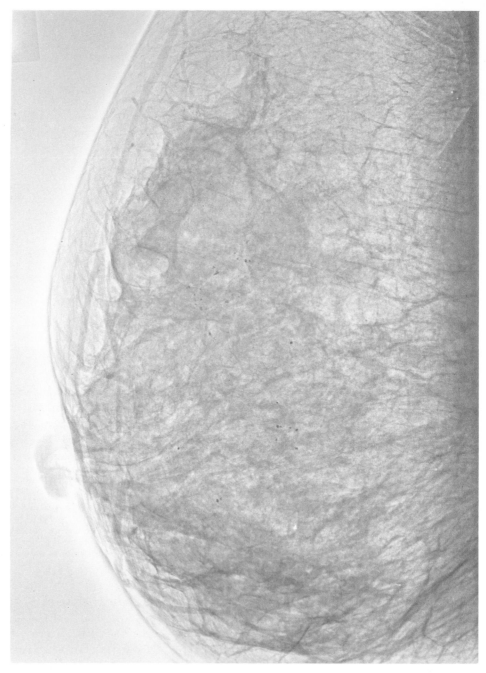

Fig. 5.4 Benign mammary dysplasia: there is uniformly dense tissue throughout the breast with scattered small round calcifications. Age 38.

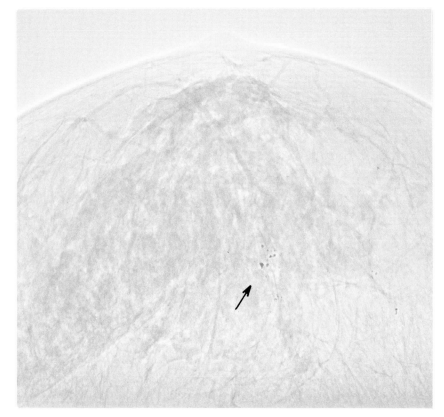

Fig. 5.5   Benign mammary dysplasia: dense tissue shown histologically to be due to BMD with areas of sclerosing adenosis. The group of calcifications (arrow) were in the walls of microcysts. Age 48.

hormonally-active patient with dense normal parenchyma. However, severe dysplastic changes of the nodular type cause such great density that the condition is diagnosable even in the young. Changes of this type are notorious for their ability to obscure localized abnormality. However, there is occasionally very poor correlation between the clinical and radiological features, clear symptoms and signs of dysplasia occurring in patients who mammographically have breasts which appear to be largely replaced by fat. Similarly, gross histological changes of benign mammary dysplasia may be found in patients with normal mammograms.

The increased density due to dysplasia is most easily recognized in the postmenopausal patient where breast parenchyma usually atrophies and is largely replaced by fat. In this age group dense tissue occupying more than just the outer quadrant usually signifies BMD. Occasionally, elderly patients will show very dense dysplastic tissue symmetrically but only distributed in a subareolar location. Biopsy will show this represents fibrosis alone, without epithelial hyperplasia.

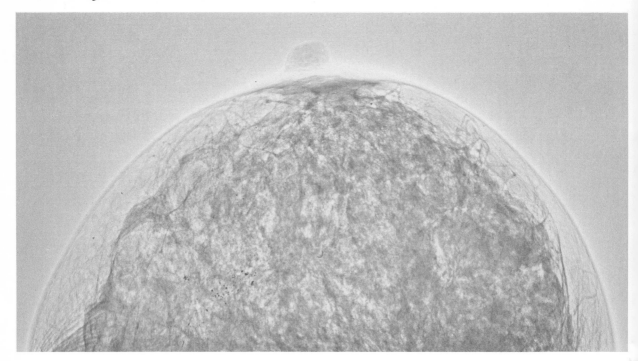

Fig. 5.6   Benign mammary dysplasia: densely nodular breast tissue containing grouped calcifications which were in fibrous tissue and in the walls of ducts. Age 50.

A localized area of very dense fibrosis with a spiculated outline and sometimes containing calcification may occur among more generalized BMD, due to sclerosing adenosis, which can be mammographically indistinguishable from carcinoma (Figs 5.2, 5.3 and 5.5). Sometimes the changes are subtle producing no more than a disturbance of the normal breast architecture. A number of features, such as the type of calcification and the distribution of the density within the abnormal area and as to whether this constitutes a central mass, have been carefully examined in an attempt to allow these two conditions to be differentiated but none have proved reliable. In these circumstances the radiologist is wise to indicate the risk of malignancy and the need for biopsy even when he considers sclerosing adenosis to be the most likely diagnosis.

Calcifications are common in BMD. They are usually found in each breast, symmetrically distributed. There may be just a small number or they may be uncountable. The calcifications are usually small, less than 0.5 mm in diameter, and round. Angular calcifications are less frequent in BMD than in carcinomas which contain calcium, and, linear calcifications are uncommon. The calcium occurs in fibrous tissue, in the walls of ducts, in inspissated secretions within ducts, or, within the walls of microcysts (Figs 5.2–5.6).

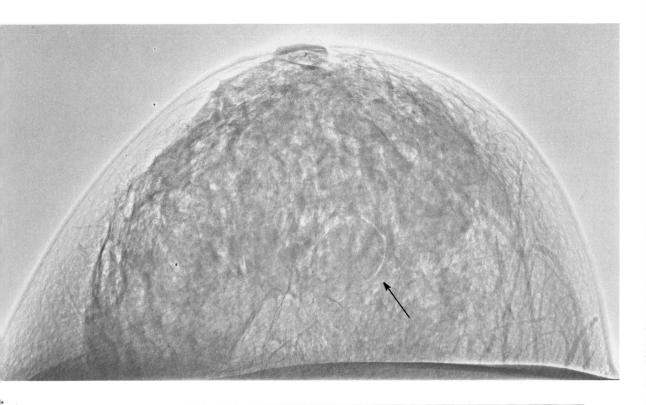

Fig. 5.7 Cyst: the well-defined round
outline of a cyst (arrow) can be
identified amongst densely dysplastic
tissue because of the surrounding halo
of fat. Age 37.

Fig. 5.8 Cyst: the breast contains a
good deal of fat revealing a P2 duct
pattern and a clear cut outline of a
cyst. Age 56. ▶

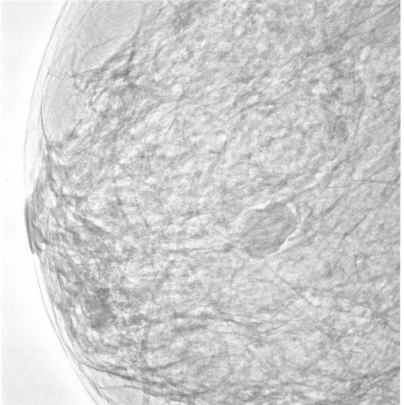

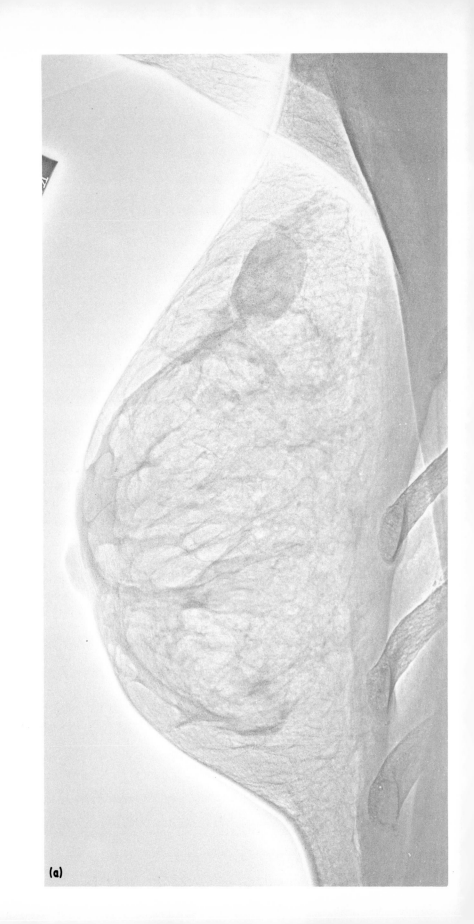

(a)

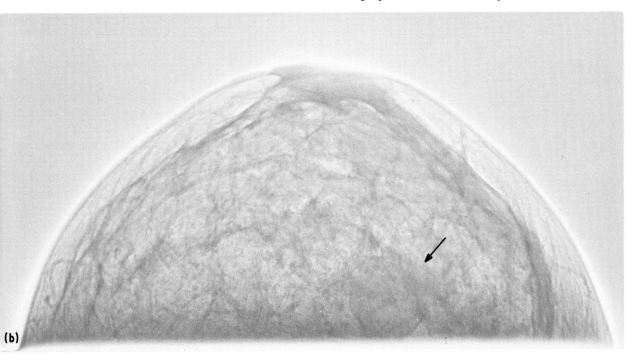

(b)

Fig. 5.9   Infected cyst: the outline of the cyst is well defined in the lateral view (a) but obscured (arrow) on the cranio-caudad projection (b). Biopsy showed the cyst was infected. Age 35.

Cysts

Radiologically demonstrable cysts are a common but not an essential component of BMD. The cysts are formed by dilatations of the lactiferous ducts and range in size from microcysts to those which occupy virtually the whole of the breast. They are usually multiple and bilateral. Even in those cases where radiologically there appears to be only a solitary cyst, multiple cysts are found at surgery. They are usually round in outline and if there is a conglomerate collection of cysts they present a lobulated outline. Cysts may accompany increased density as a result of the other components of BMD (Fig. 5.7) or the remaining breast may be of normal density (Fig. 5.8). In the latter case the whole of the cyst outline can be clearly visualized but that may not be the case when fibrous tissue or adenosis are present and lie immediately against the cyst, so that part of the silhouette is lost. Early authors described loss of part of an otherwise well-defined outline as a feature of malignant change but failure to identify part of the cyst outline is so common that this becomes a useless sign. When the cyst outline can be identified it is usually sharply defined (Fig. 5.9). In very dense breasts the outline may not be identifiable at all and the presence of a cyst is recognized solely as an additional density (Fig. 5.10). In these cases it is essential for needle aspiration to be undertaken to confirm the lesion as a cyst.

Differential diagnosis of cyst from fibroadenoma or an unusually well-circumscribed carcinoma such as a medullary tumour may be impossible on radiological grounds alone. Therefore needle aspiration of solitary cysts should be a routine part of the examination. Other helpful features in diagnosing the lesions as cysts are their ultrasonic characteristics, multiplicity and patient age. Multiple cysts are very much more common than multiple fibroadenomas (Fig. 5.11). Cysts are unusual before the age of 25 when fibroadenomas are most common, and cysts are rarely seen after the menopause. However, fibroadenomas which form in the patient's early twenties may remain unchanged and uncalcified until after the menopause. A halo of compressed fat may be seen around any longstanding firm lesion and so is not a helpful differentiating feature.

Two types of calcification occur in the walls of cysts (Fig. 5.12). Microcysts may contain two or three small round calcifications, indeed, these may be the only abnormalities on the mammogram. A histological diagnosis of cystic disease is then an unexpected finding following biopsy. Larger cysts may contain fine curvilinear mural calcifications which are only demonstrable in the surfaces of the cyst that are tangential to the X-ray beam.

Although needle aspiration plays an important role in the diagnosis of cysts, we do not feel that cystography should be used as a routine. The best indications for cystography are a bloody aspirate, a mass remaining after cyst aspiration and early refilling. Tumours arising within cysts are so uncommon that routine cystography would be an unrewarding exercise. However, cysts and carcinomas are such common pathologies that they are often found in the same breast. The radiologist must not allow his attention to be fully occupied by an obvious cyst and risk missing a small carcinoma elsewhere in the breast.

Cysts fluctuate in size throughout the menstrual cycle and may contribute to premenstrual discomfort. There are similar changes in size over longer intervals so that serial examinations may show one cyst decreasing in size as another increases.

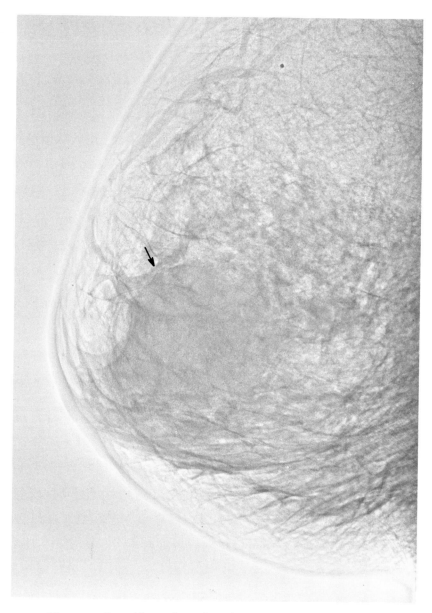

Fig. 5.10 Cyst: this cyst is causing a homogeneous area of increased density
with generally poorly-defined margins except for the antero-superior surface
(arrow). Age 55.

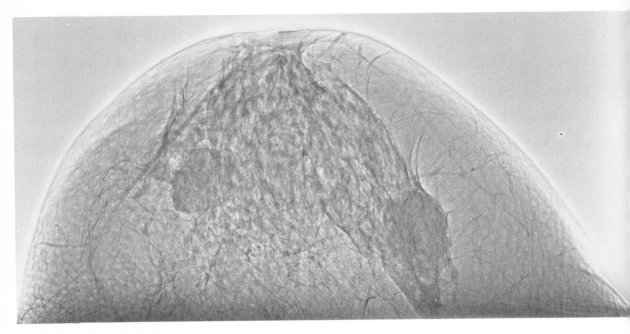

Fig. 5.11 Cysts: there is a P2 duct
pattern with two well-defined masses.
No fluid was obtained at needle
aspiration. Biopsy revealed very thick-
walled cysts and gross surrounding
fibrosis. Age 52.

Fig. 5.12 Cyst calcification: punctate calcifications (arrow) were present in the
wall of a small cyst (a) and curvilinear mural calcification in one of a
collection of cysts (b). ▶

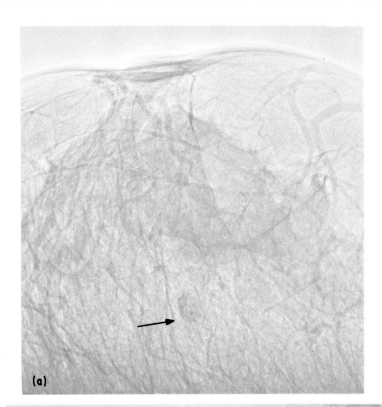

(a)

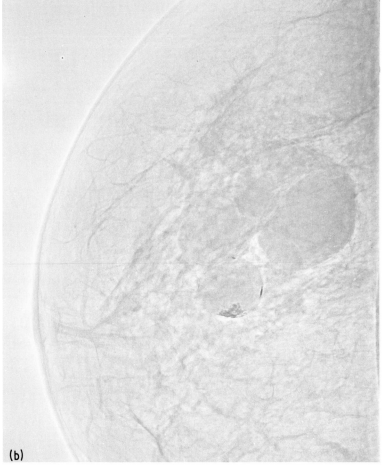

(b)

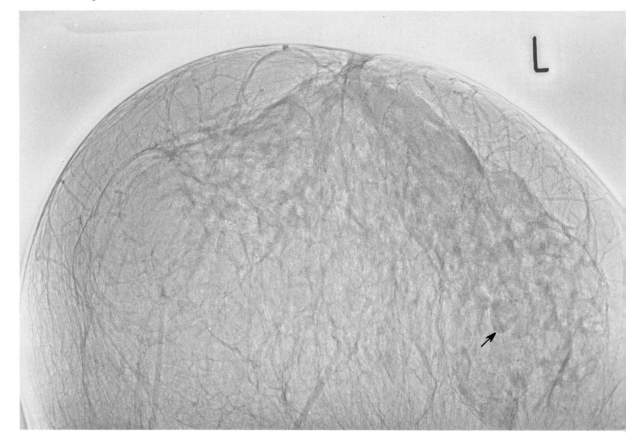

Fig. 5.13   Normal lymph node: the small well-defined opacity (arrow) in the upper outer quadrant of a 62-year-old patient is a lymph node. The adjacent breast tissue is dense due to BMD. Bilateral chains of lymph nodes are recognizable for what they are, but, solitary nodes may be indistinguishable from a cyst or fibroadenoma.

Ductal abnormalities

The ductal changes associated with BMD involve both the epithelium and the duct wall. Hyperplasia of the epithelium may be so profuse that it becomes folded, this is described as papillomatosis. In the wall proliferation of myoepithelial cells and periductal collagenosis cause an increase in the size and density of the ducts which then appear beaded and nodular on the mammogram (Figs 5.14 and 5.15). The epithelial changes may obstruct the duct and cause its distension by retained secretions. Dilatation of a single duct is an important radiological observation as it may also be caused by an obstructing proximal tumour or by a deep tumour permeating forward to the nipple along the duct.

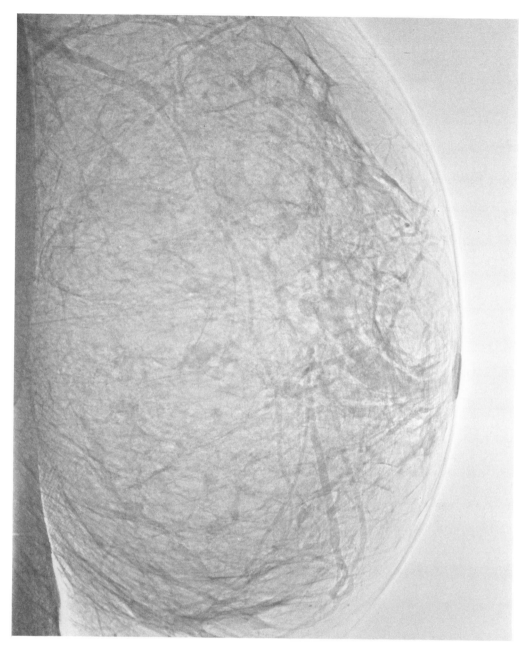

Fig. 5.14 Papillomatosis: dilated ducts immediately deep to the nipple due to the profound epithelial hyperplasia which is described as papillomatosis.

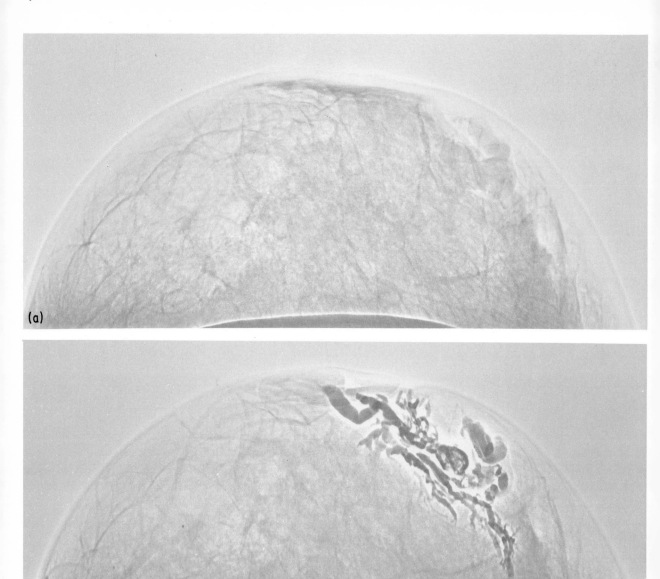

(a)

(b)

Fig. 5.15 Papillomatosis: a dilated tortuous duct obstructed by
papillomatosis shown on plain film (a) and ductogram (b).

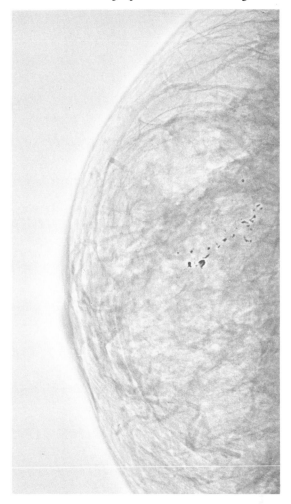

Fig. 5.16   Papillomatosis: quite large calcifications of various shapes lie in the line of a duct. Whilst papillomatosis is the most likely diagnosis intraduct carcinoma cannot be excluded radiologically.

Periductal collagenosis is often hidden by the density of the surrounding parenchyma in premenopausal patients but becomes evident as the density decreases with advancing years.

Calcifications may occur along the course of a duct particularly in the presence of papillomatosis. There are usually rather a small number, less than 10, with a round smooth outline. Whilst small calcifications, less than 0.5 mm in diameter, are most common they are occasionally 1–2 mm in diameter. Even then it is impossible to be sure that they represent papillomatosis since similar calcification can be found in intraduct carcinoma (Figs 5.16–5.18). In rare cases papillomatosis produces an irregular area of increased density containing calcification.

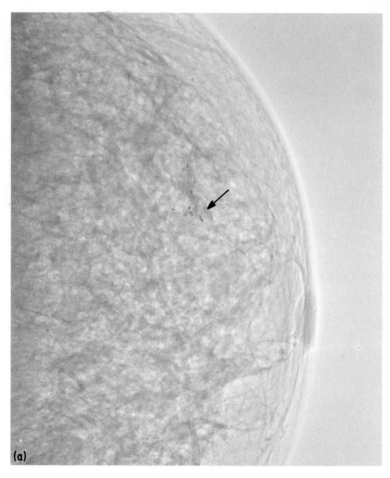

(a)

Fig. 5.17 Papillomatosis: the soft tissue density of a dilated duct (arrow) is accompanied by a number of small round calcifications running in the same direction.

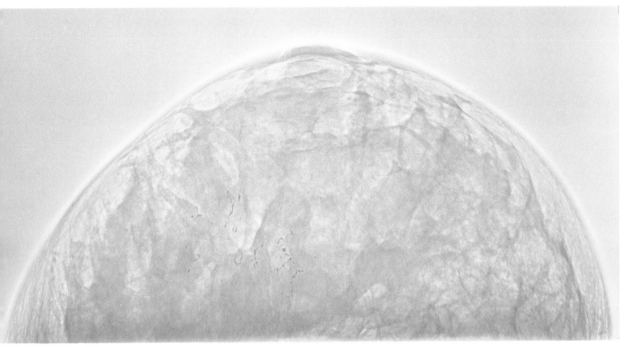

Fig. 5.18 Papillomatosis: very unusually grouped linear calcification due to papillomatosis. These appearances are much more frequently associated with carcinoma.

SECRETORY DISEASE

Secretory disease is a term which embraces the pathological features of duct ectasia and the associated clinical signs which include nipple discharge and retraction. The condition is common and is seen in patients aged 30 onwards. There may be no symptoms for years so that the precise age of onset is difficult to determine. The condition is usually bilateral and it is characterized by obstructed ducts, due to epithelial hyperplasia, with associated proximal dilatation which may be cystic. The dilated tortuous beaded ducts are often, but not always, visible on the mammogram particularly in a subareolar location. The bilateral nature of the condition helps in its diagnosis.

Calcification within inspissated secretions and within the duct walls are common and have a characteristic appearance, often being either tubular or circular with a lucent centre (Figs 5.19–5.21). Most of the calcifications are greater than 1 mm in diameter and they are often a good deal larger. The intraductal position can be recognized by the branching format of some of the linear calcifications.

Nipple retraction is often evident on the mammogram. After congenital retraction, secretory disease is the second most common cause of

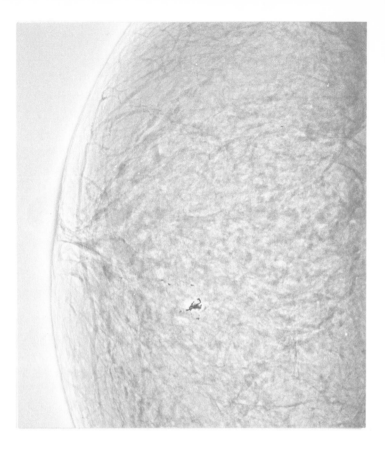

Fig. 5.19   Secretory disease: bizarre calcification which was found to lie in the walls of dilated ducts which were surrounded by fibrous tissue.

longstanding bilateral nipple retraction. Care must be taken to exclude evidence of malignancy deep to the nipple, particularly when this sign is unilateral. There is no skin thickening of the areola in this condition which can be a helpful differential point.

Plasma cell mastitis

Plasma cell mastitis is a common complication of secretory disease and represents an inflammatory response, usually chronic, to secretions escaping through a duct wall into the surrounding tissue. Radiologically one sees an ill-defined area of increased density deep to the nipple associated with signs of secretory disease in a patient with clinical features of inflammation (Fig. 5.22).

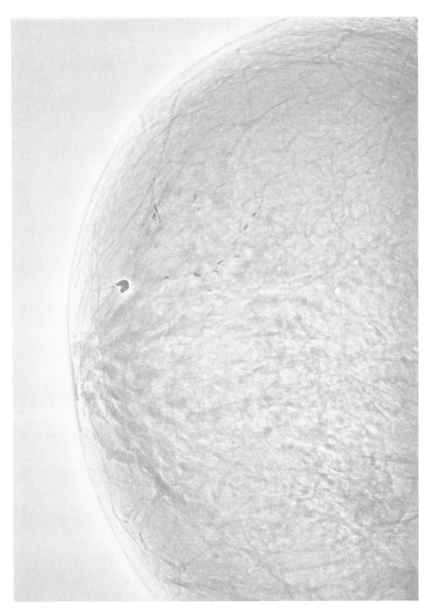

Fig. 5.20 Secretory disease: there are prominent ducts some of which contain broad linear calcifications.

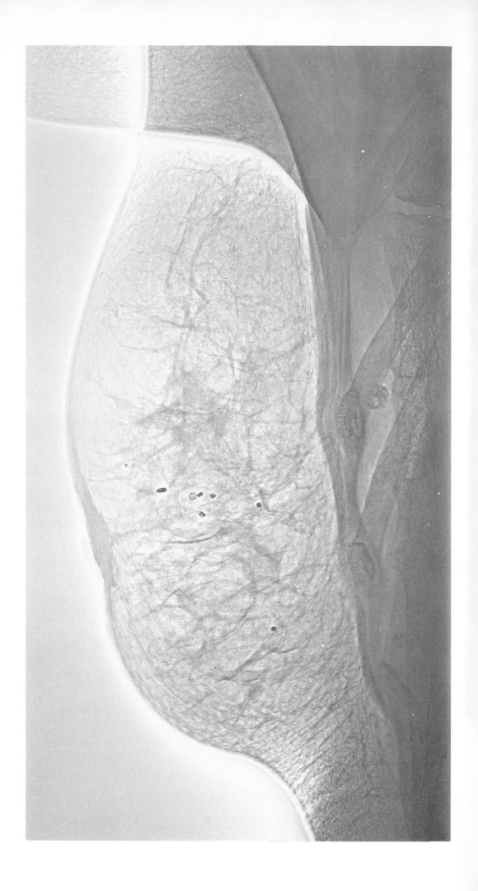

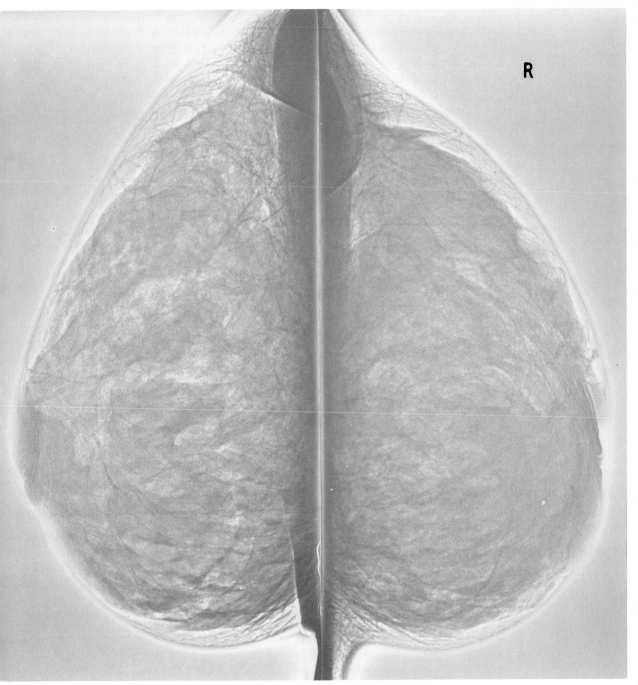

R

▲ Fig. 5.22 Plasma cell mastitis: diffuse increased density is present deep to the retracted right nipple. Histology showed chronic inflammatory changes with plasma cells predominant.

◄ Fig. 5.21 Secretory disease: round calcifications with lucent centres lie within ectatic ducts. The nipple is slightly retracted.

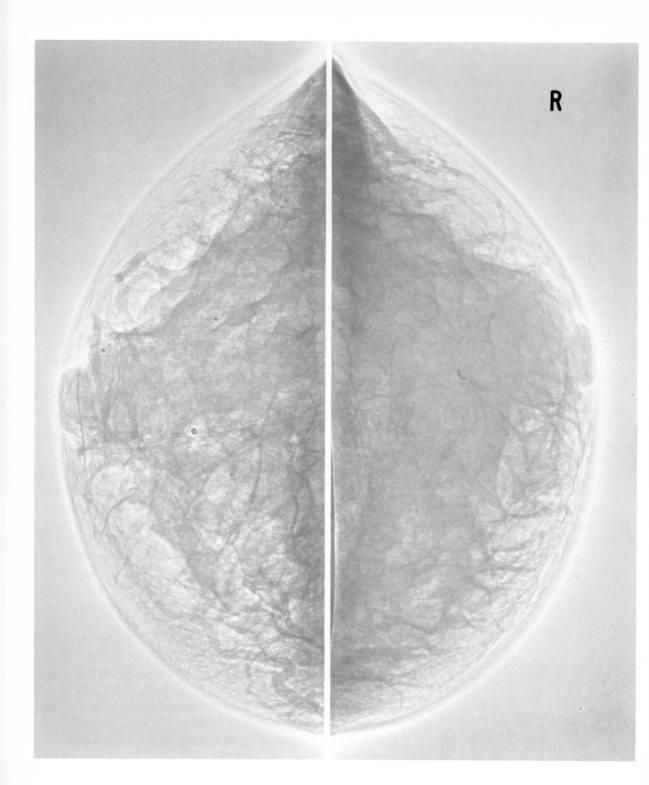

R

ACUTE MASTITIS AND ABSCESS

Most acute inflammations of the breast, whether frank abscess formation takes place or not, occur during lactation. The symptoms and physical signs are usually obvious and respond to antibiotics and, when necessary, surgical drainage. In these circumstances, mammography is rarely required. During lactation the breast parenchyma is extremely dense so that abnormalities due to acute mastitis may be difficult to demonstrate.

Acute inflammatory changes due to infection occurring in the absence of lactation are much less common. The important diagnostic problem is to differentiate inflammatory signs associated with infection from those associated with carcinoma. Both conditions produce an ill-defined increase in density usually involving a large area and often the whole breast. Inflammatory oedema may cause thickening of the supporting trabeculae and of the skin (Fig. 5.23). This is most often seen in the area overlying the inflamed breast tissue but may be accompanied by thickening of the most dependent part of the breast or of the whole breast. There is often increased vascularity compared with the opposite side and enlarged axillary and intramammary lymph nodes.

The similarity of the two conditions may not allow their differentiation by mammography at the initial examination. Needle aspiration for cytology will provide the diagnosis at that time. Where this technique is not available, response to antibiotics can be recorded by mammography but it usually takes three or four weeks for the inflammatory signs to settle to any noticeable degree.

Occasionally cysts become infected and show no mammographic features other than the well-defined mass of the cyst with few or no signs of inflammation in the surrounding tissues (Fig. 5.10).

BENIGN TUMOURS

Fibroadenoma

Fibroadenomas are often very easy to feel but difficult to see. These benign tumours occur most commonly before age 30, with the peak incidence at 20–25 years, when the breast parenchyma is most dense. The whole or part of the lesion may be obscured by the surrounding breast tissue (Fig. 5.24). When visible, the outline is well defined and round or lobulated and may be surrounded by a halo of fat (Fig. 5.25). Fibroadenomas are usually single but occasionally there are two or three and rarely many are present simultaneously (Figs 5.26 and 5.27). The size usually lies within the range 0.5–5 cm. Clinically there is cyclical variation in size but this is not usually

Fig. 5.23   Abscess: there is increased density centrally on the right with skin thickening. No increase in vascularity is apparent.

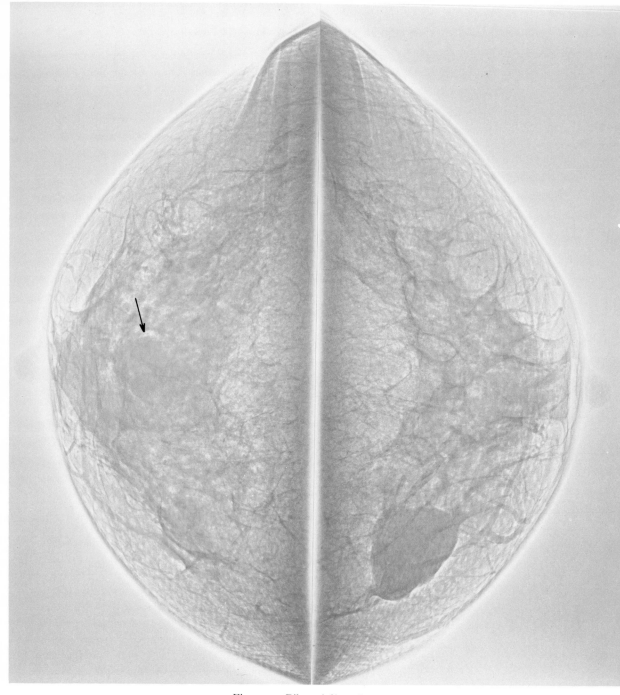

Fig. 5.24 Bilateral fibroadenoma: a well-defined lobulated mass is shown on the right but the fibroadenoma on the left is partly obscured by surrounding dense tissue (arrow). Age 33.

Fig. 5.25 Fibroadenoma: a well-defined round mass with a surrounding halo of fat. The adjacent breast tissue is slightly greater in density than elsewhere in that breast, histology showed the fibroadenoma lying in an area of BMD. Age 45. ▶

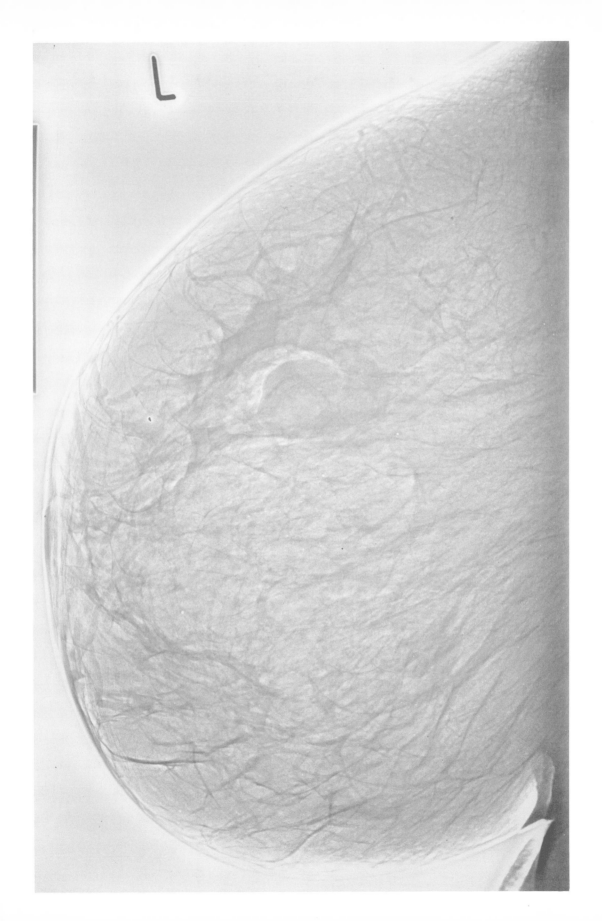

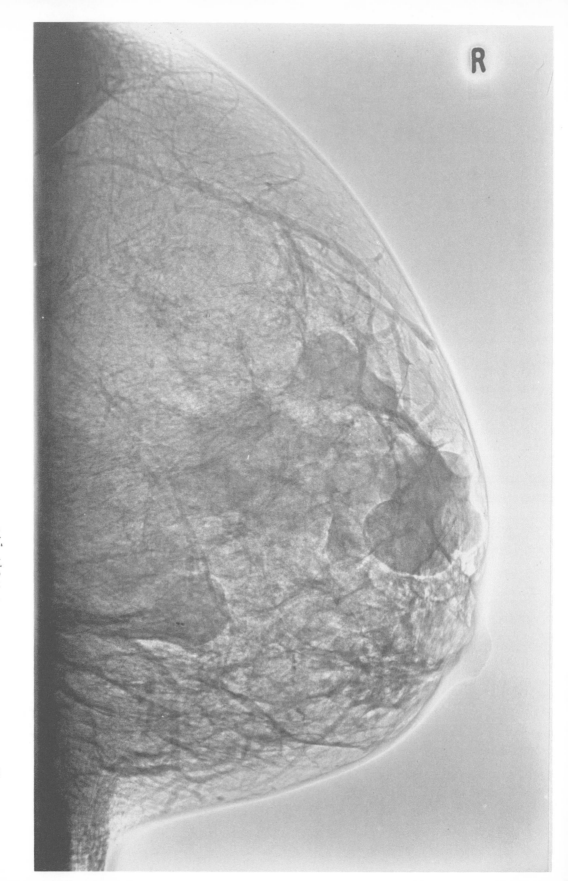

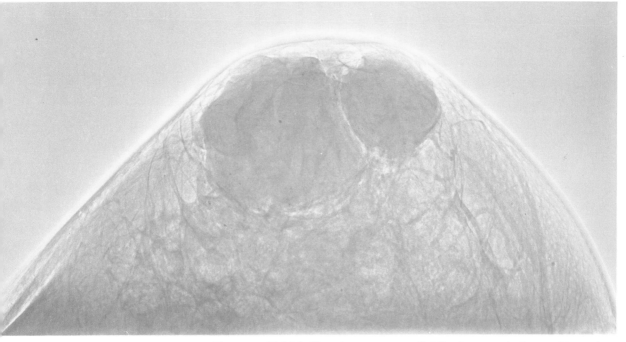

Fig. 5.27 Multiple fibroadenomas: two well-defined masses, the larger with a craggy outline. Histology showed fibroadenomas. Multiple calcifications are present in the surrounding dysplastic tissue.

◄
Fig. 5.26 Multiple fibroadenomas: multiple well-defined masses some of which had increased in size during two years of follow-up. The deepest lesion contains two calcifications. Histology fibroadenoma. Age 30.

Fig. 5.28 Calcified fibroadenoma: the large plaques of calcium are characteristic of a degenerated fibroadenoma. ►

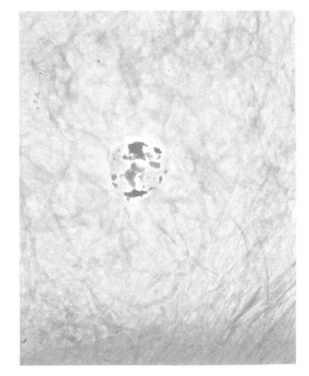

EAST GLAMORGAN HOSPITAL.
CHURCH VILLAGE. near PONTYPRIDD

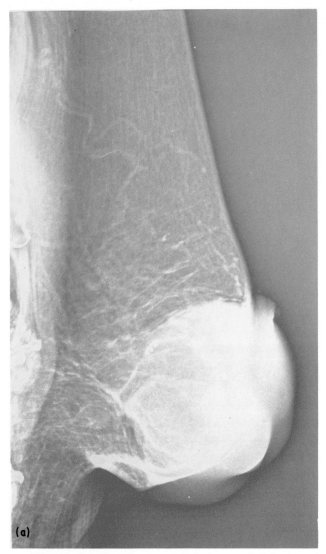

(a)

Fig. 5.29 Bilateral giant fibroadenomas: (a) the large well-defined opacity protruding through the skin is a giant fibroadenoma (cystosarcoma phylloides) and there is another similar but smaller tumour in the opposite breast (b). Age 72.

evident radiologically. However, considerable increase in size may occur during pregnancy and lactation. Longstanding fibroadenomas regress in size as the patient becomes menopausal. Cystic change or myxoid degeneration often occur in these longstanding tumours but this is not evident radiologically. They do however often calcify. This typically takes the form of very large plaques often predominantly in the periphery of the lesion, but, is also seen scattered throughout the body of the tumour. The

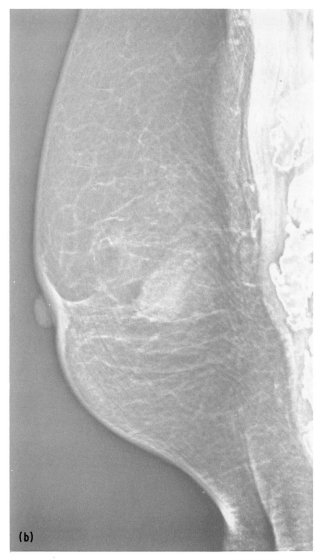

(b)

Fig. 5.29

large calcifications are usually so characteristic that the lesion can be diagnosed with absolute certainty (Fig. 5.28).

Fibroadenomas, having both epithelial and mesodermal components, have the potential for both carcinomatous and sarcomatous change and very rarely this does occur. The radiological evidence is irregularity in outline and extension into the adjacent tissues. Whilst the sharp outline of a fibroadenoma is usually very good evidence of benignicity just occasionally carcinomas have identical features. It is therefore a wise policy to excise all such lesions which are solitary, even if needle aspiration

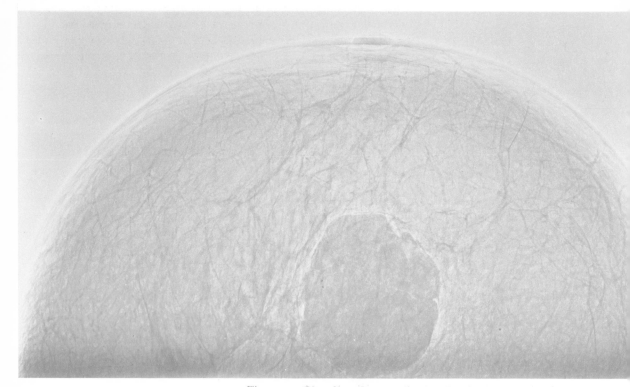

Fig. 5.30   Giant fibroadenoma: a large well-defined lobulated mass containing only two calcifications. Histology showed the leaf-like (phylloides) cellular pattern of giant fibroadenoma. No evidence of malignancy. Age 63.

for cytology reveals cells characteristic of fibroadenoma, since malignant change developing elsewhere within the lesion cannot altogether be excluded.

Giant fibroadenoma

This condition is much less frequent than the fibroadenoma discussed above and is found predominantly in middle-aged women although occasional cases are found in adolescence and also after the menopause. The term cystosarcoma phylloides has been used previously but as there is no primary relationship with sarcoma this name should be avoided. However sarcomatous and carcinomatous change can occur as in the standard form of fibroadenoma and very rarely the tumour metastisizes.

Since giant fibroadenomas occur in the middle-aged where fatty replacement of breast tissue has commonly taken place there is usually no difficulty in identifying the smooth, roughly rounded outline of the tumour. They are mainly solitary but may be multiple (Fig. 5.29). The lesion is usually large by the time the patient presents and may involve virtually the whole breast and may even stretch and thin the skin. Calcification can occur within the mass but it is much less frequent than in the ordinary fibroadenoma and when it does occur is usually not very great in degree (Fig. 5.30). These tumours recur locally if excision is incomplete so that a postoperative mammogram may be helpful.

Duct papilloma

Duct papilloma which is usually a solitary benign tumour must be differentiated from papillomatosis which is a descriptive term for a profuse form of epithelial hyperplasia. A duct papilloma is recognized as a well-defined round or lobulated mass usually 0.5–2 cm in diameter lying close to the nipple. As the papilloma enlarges its shape may be determined by the confining walls of the duct so that it may take on a more finger-like shape. In addition the obstructed duct may become distended by retained secretions. The abnormality is usually easily identified but may be obscured by the opacity caused by normal ducts converging at the nipple. Exactly similar findings may be due to intraduct carcinoma, so that excision biopsy should be advised. Galactography may be helpful in identifying the pathological duct.

Lipoma

Lipomas are not uncommon in postmenopausal patients. This may be an incidental radiological finding in a patient with no clinical symptoms or signs or there may be a well-defined mass in which the patient has noticed no change for years. The diagnosis is made by the identification of a fine smooth capsule surrounding an area of low density fat (Figs 5.31 and 5.32). Occasionally septa can be identified passing from one side of the capsule to the other. Lipomas vary in size from 1–2 cm to huge lesions displacing the normal breast parenchyma. Occasionally patients are seen in which the distribution of fat is obviously asymmetric when the two breasts are compared but with no capsule formation. Fat of this type can also have a mass effect displacing the normal parenchyma.

TRAUMA

Haematoma

Haematomas can occur spontaneously in the breast but usually follow trauma. Needle aspiration commonly causes some bleeding so that this test should always be carried out after rather than before mammography as the blood may obscure the primary pathology, or add features which lead to misinterpretation. It is, of course, essential that the radiologist is made aware of the history of trauma.

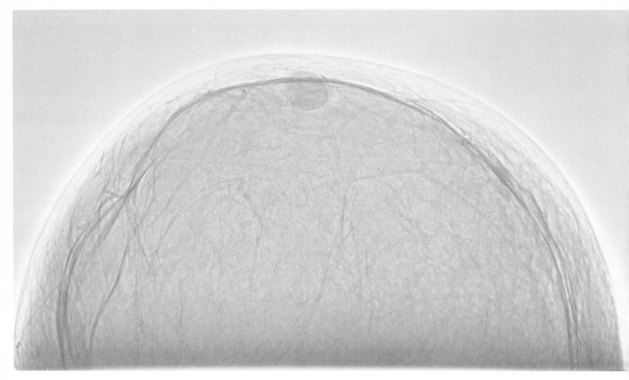

Fig. 5.31   Lipoma: the most obvious feature of this low density lipoma is the surrounding capsule.

The evidence of haematoma depends upon its size. A small haemorrhage causes an ill-defined area of increased density which is often nodular and within which the normal trabeculae appear distorted. The overlying skin may be thickened (Fig. 5.33). Larger haematomas are occasionally seen following excisional surgery. The blood-filled operative cavity produces a well-defined but irregular opacity which is very dense for its size. The lesion decreases in size over a week or two except rarely when an organized haematoma forms a lasting mass.

Fat necrosis

Fat necrosis is most often found in the large fatty postmenopausal breast where it produces changes which may mimic cancer. Trauma, including previous surgery, is the most common aetiology or the condition can follow an inflammatory process, but, there may be no such predisposing

Fig. 5.32   Lipoma: a rounded capsule surrounds low density fat. The soft tissue densities overlying the lesion are in compressed adjacent normal tissue.

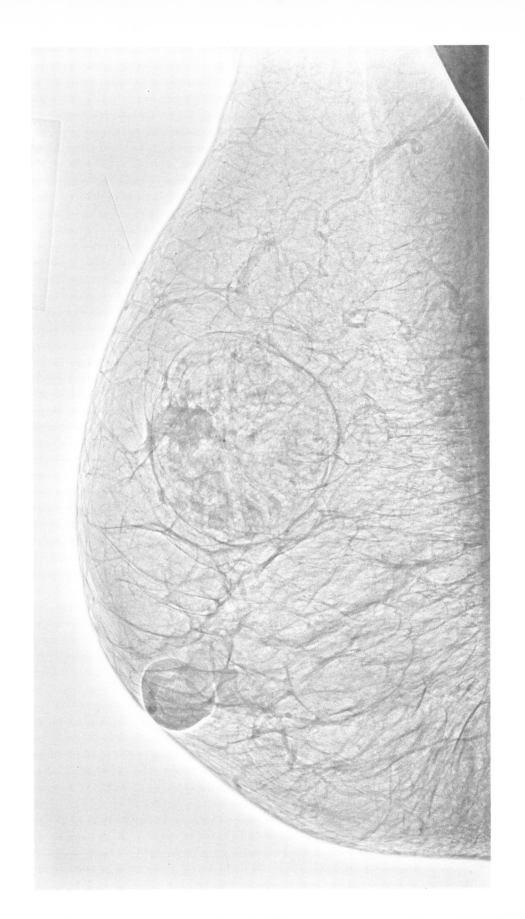

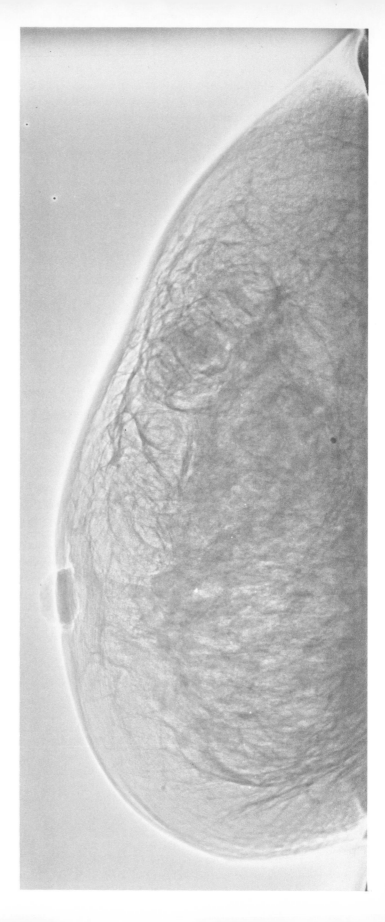

Fig. 5.33   Haematoma: following
needle aspiration there is increased
density and distortion of the
subcutaneous structures and skin
thickening, due to bleeding.

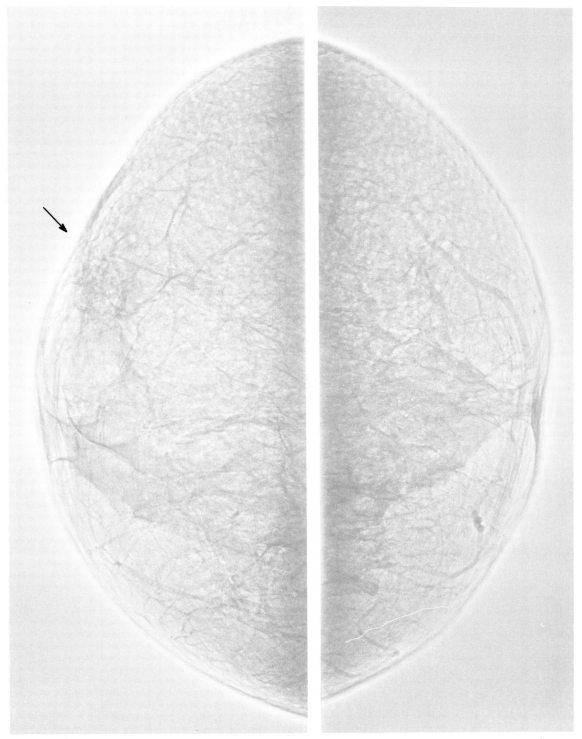

Fig. 5.34 Fat necrosis: four weeks after a seat belt injury there is increased density and distortion of the subcutaneous tissue with skin retraction (arrow). Biopsy showed fat necrosis.

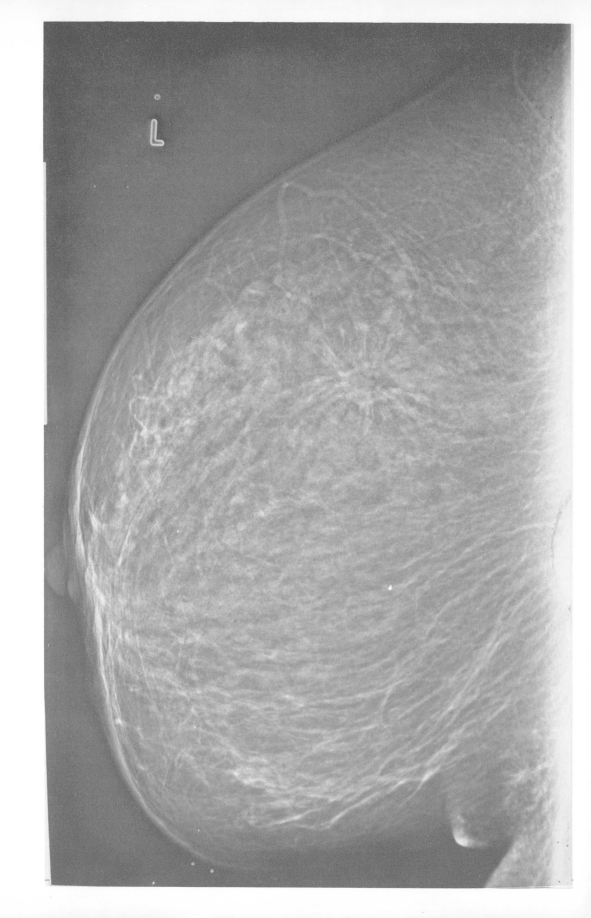

Fig. 5.35 Fat necrosis: the patient presented with a mass and skin retraction. Mammography shows a spiculated mass thought to be a carcinoma. Biopsy revealed fat necrosis only.

circumstance. The most frequent mammographic abnormality is a spiculated mass which may contain calcification (Fig. 5.34). There may be overlying skin thickening or retraction so that differentiation from cancer may be impossible from the mammogram alone (Fig. 5.35).

Fat necrosis is occasionally an unexpected histological finding in a patient with typical mammographic features of benign mammary dysplasia. Calcification can be the only radiological abnormality and may have a characteristic ring format. The ring-shaped calcifications surround 'oil cysts' (Fig. 5.36). These may be seen in operation cavities or in the subcutaneous fat following an abscess. The most striking examples are seen associated with acne usually involving the inframammary fold or the most medial part of the breast. Ring calcifications are usually multiple and may be 2–3 mm in diameter or as large as 1 cm.

Scarring

Cooperation from referring clinicians in indicating the site of previous operations is vitally important to the radiologist. The radiographers must also be trained to look for scars so that a double check is made. Scarring can cause changes so like carcinoma that the radiologist will be repeatedly caught out if this information is not available.

Fig. 5.36 Oil cysts: ring calcifications were present throughout the subcutaneous fat in the lower part of each breast in a patient with longstanding and gross acne. The oil cysts are areas of fat necrosis following inflammation.

Even extremely well-healed small scars cause localized skin thickening with a linear opacity due to fibrosis passing into the subcutaneous fat. If the excised volume of breast tissue was large there may be enough fibrosis

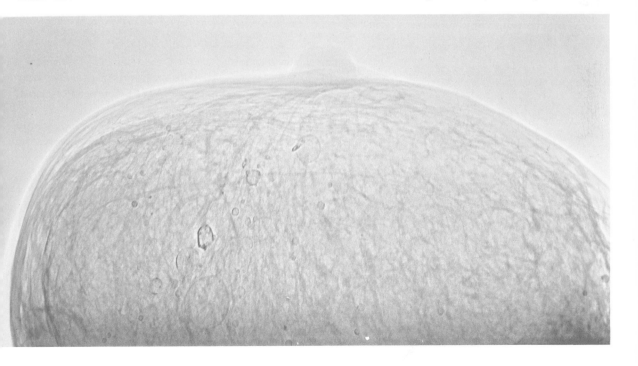

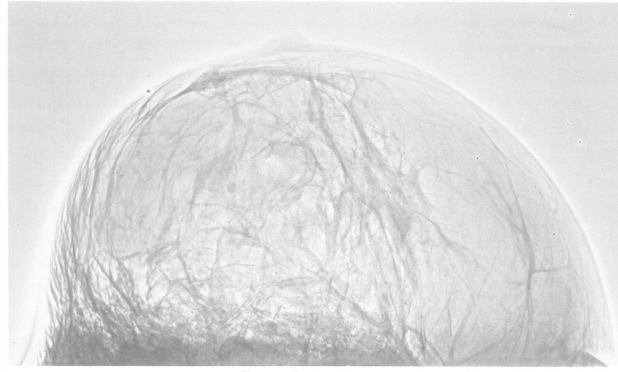

Fig. 5.37   Scarring: the breast tissue is distorted due to a reduction mammoplasty.

to cause a spiculated mass with associated skin retraction. If this occurs centrally the nipple may retract. A mammogram taken in the early postoperative follow-up period is invaluable as a baseline against which to measure later enlarging masses (Fig. 5.37).

When there is no direct mammographic evidence of scarring the only change due to previous surgery may be the lack of symmetry between the two breasts due to the removal of tissue. Whenever there is asymmetry one should look for a history of previous biopsy on the less dense side.

Considerable difficulty can occur in recognizing tumour arising in a breast scarred by previous surgery. The difficulty centres around deciding which abnormal features one can deduct from the mammogram as being due to the previous surgery. It is then helpful to have the position of skin scars identified by having fine wire attached to the breast prior to mammography. Unfortunately the skin incision does not always give a precise indication of the extent of dissection in the breast tissue. When differentiation between scarring and cancer is proving difficult needle aspiration of the suspicious area, possibly using mammography control, may be needed.

Calcifications may develop within scar tissue deep within the breast or in the skin, particularly if there is keloid formation when the calcifications are usually coarse and linear sometimes producing a network (Fig. 5.38). Within scarred breast parenchyma calcifications are small and usually rounded but may be linear. They may occur alone or accompany increased density due to fibrosis. In these circumstances it can be very difficult to rule out cancer. The calcifications lie within thrombosed vessels, areas of fat necrosis, fibrous tissue and in foreign body granulomas around suture material.

Occasionally after axillary dissection generalized lymphoedema occurs causing skin thickening particularly in the most dependent part of the breast and a generalized increase in density due to oedema throughout the parenchyma.

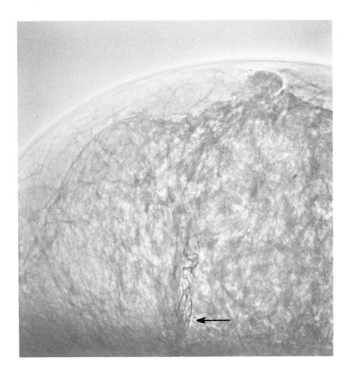

Fig. 5.38   Scar calcification: lattice-like calcification (arrow) in a keloid scar.

6 MAMMOGRAPHIC FEATURES OF MALIGNANCY

C.A. Parsons

There are few techniques which offer the radiologist a greater opportunity to help cancer patients than mammography. Many radiological investigations have an important part to play in establishing a diagnosis or defining the extent of disease but few influence the patient's prognosis as favourably as the detection of 'early' curable breast cancer. Unfortunately, the converse is also true that failure to recognize mammographic signs of clinically occult breast cancer can change the patient's prognosis from 100% five year survival to the poor outlook, 40% five year survival, found in patients presenting with symptomatic disease.

All radiological techniques have their limitations. Even first class mammography will fail to show about 10% of tumours. Half of these will be obscured by the increased density of benign mammary dysplasia or the density of normal glandular tissue in the younger patient and the other half are not shown even in fatty atrophic breasts. This is due simply to this group of tumours having similar attenuating properties to normal breast tissue. We have to rely on other modalities, such as clinical examination or ultrasound, for their detection. This situation is captured in the dictum that 'bad news from the radiologist is usually valid but good news is not much better than no news'. Mammographic suspicion of carcinoma is as much an indication for breast biopsy as suspicious clinical findings. However, in the face of suspicious physical signs a negative mammogram should be overlooked.

The most important role of mammography in breast cancer is undoubtedly the detection of clinically occult disease but, outside of screening projects, this is a relatively uncommon event. More frequent roles are:

1. Identifying a benign cause for symptoms.
2. Confirmation of clinical signs of cancer.
3. Demonstration of unsuspected multicentric or bilateral tumour.
4. Monitoring response to non-surgical treatment.
5. Routine screening for recurrence.

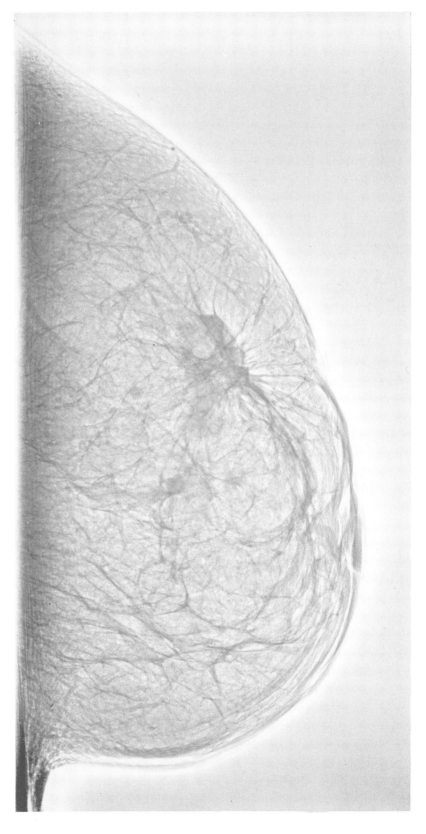

Fig. 6.1 Positive mode lateral xeromammogram showing a spiculated carcinoma causing skin retraction in a fatty N1 breast.

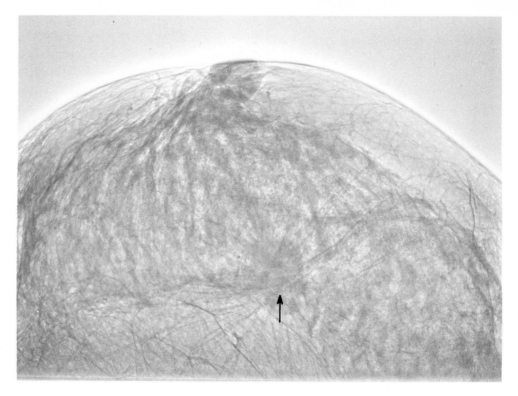

Fig. 6.2   A spiculated carcinoma (arrow) in a breast with a prominent P2 duct pattern.

There is considerable variety in the mammographic signs of malignancy due to the range of histological types of tumour, growth rate, position within the breast and the type of surrounding breast parenchyma. The evidence of malignancy can be divided into those signs which are directly due to the tumour itself and those which are caused by the effect of the tumour on its surroundings.

DIRECT EVIDENCE OF MALIGNANCY

Increased density

The most fundamental change caused by a breast tumour is increase in density compared with the surrounding normal tissue. This is caused by a number of factors. Firstly there is an increase in the number of cells per unit volume mostly due to proliferation of tumour cells but with a small contribution from host cells. Oedema may occur in the surrounding tissue contributing to the increase in density and causing haziness of outline, and, some tumours particularly the common infiltrating ductal lesions

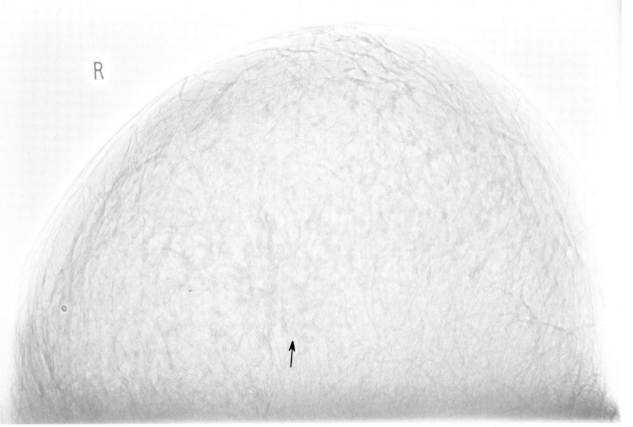

Fig. 6.3   A large spiculated tumour (arrow) of relatively low density lies centrally within the breast.

may be associated with the formation of considerable amounts of fibrous tissue in the surrounding parenchyma (Figs 6.1–6.3).

The ease with which increased density can be recognized depends upon the density of the surrounding tissue (Figs 6.4–6.6). Breast parenchyma is often extremely dense in young, hormonally-active patients particularly the nulliparous and may easily obscure a tumour mass, the same is true of the fibrotic changes which are part of benign mammary dysplasia. The majority of tumours occur in the upper outer quadrant which is the last area to lose breast tissue as it atrophies in the normal process of aging. The density caused by this residual breast tissue makes detection of tumour in this area less easy than in the inner quadrants where fatty replacement is more frequent. The same problem arises in the subareolar area where a tumour may be obscured by the opacity caused by the convergence of ducts surrounded by fibrous tissue.

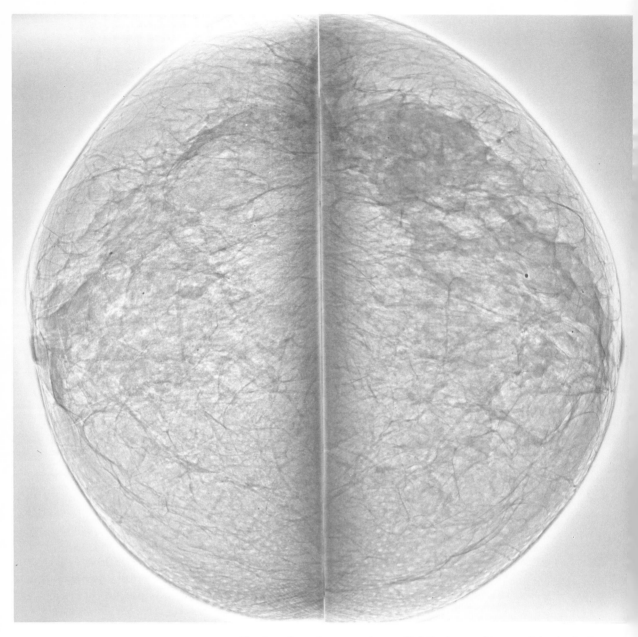

Fig. 6.4 A carcinoma causing an ill-defined area of increased density in the outer part of the breast best appreciated by comparison with the same area on the opposite side.

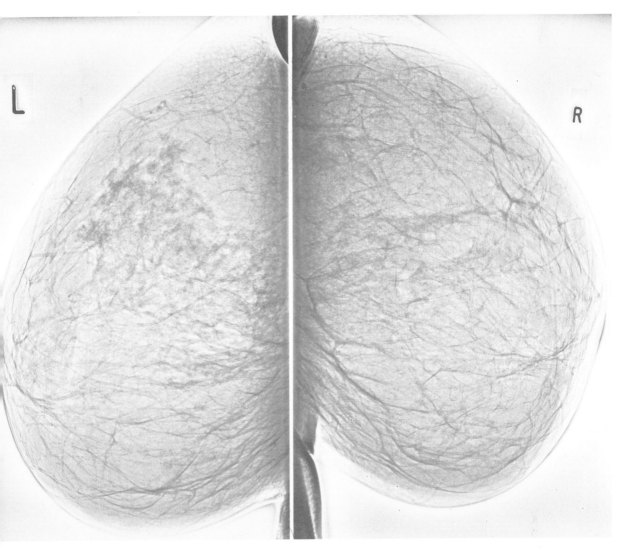

Fig. 6.5   A carcinoma causing an extremely vague ill-defined area of increased density in the upper part of the left breast.

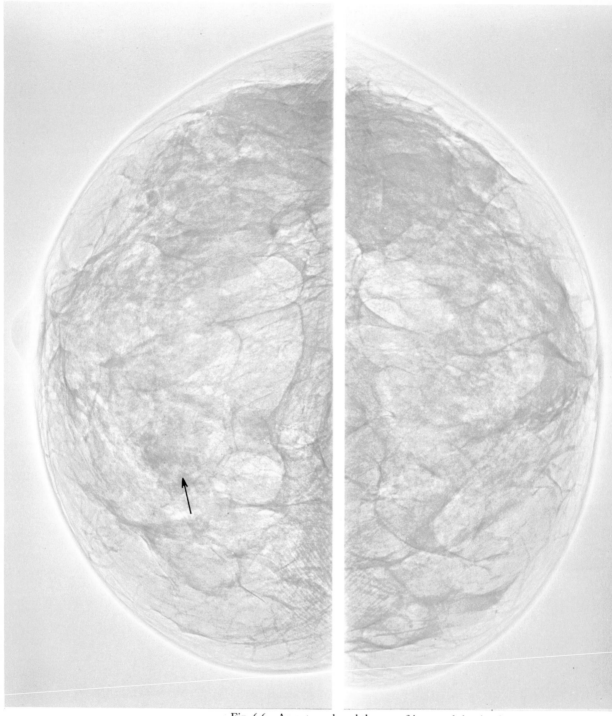

Fig. 6.6   An extremely subtle area of increased density due to tumour which would almost certainly be missed unless comparison is made with the same area of the opposite breast.

Fig. 6.7   An inflammatory carcinoma causing an overall increase in density with skin thickening and increased vascularity. ▶

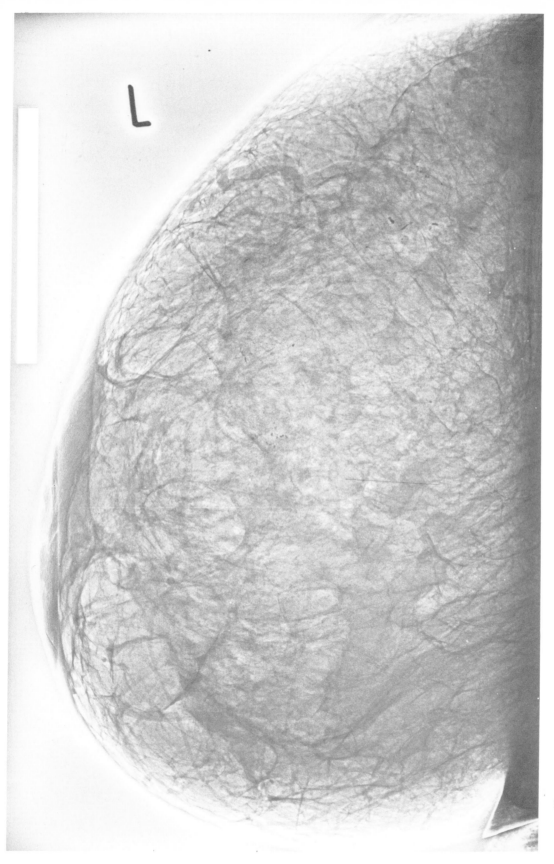

L

149

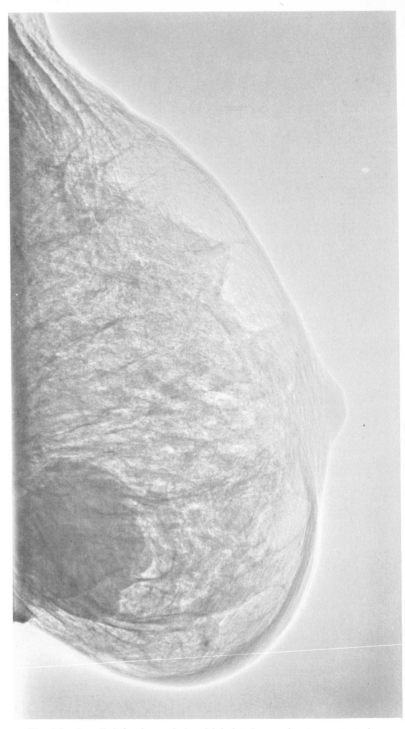

Fig. 6.8   A well–defined rounded and lobulated mass due to a metastasis from carcinoma of the uterus.

Fig. 6.9   A huge well–defined lobulated mesenchymal sarcoma occupying the lower half of the breast displacing the normal parenchyma upward. ▶

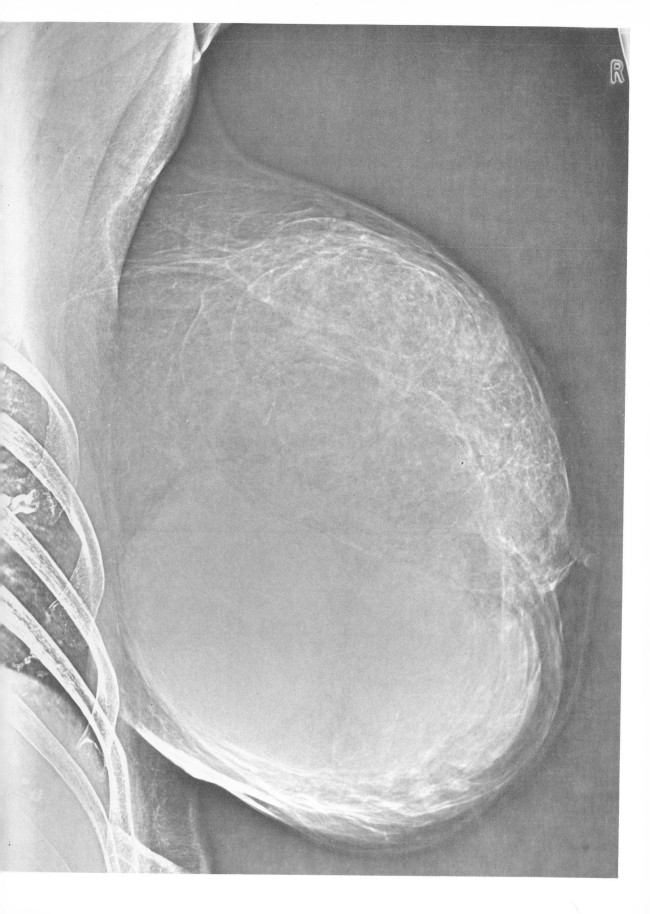

The most profound density change is seen in the uncommon inflammatory tumours (Fig. 6.7). These account for only 2% of all malignant breast tumours and are characterized by extremely rapid growth with dense infiltration over a wide area so that no boundary for the tumour can be recognized. They are commonly accompanied by skin thickening caused by direct tumour invasion or by permeation along the subdermal lymphatics causing cutaneous lymphoedema. The final factor causing increased density in these tumours is a tremendous increase in vascularity. Anderson (1980) found these very aggressive tumours usually occurred in patients in the 4th decade well before the peak incidence of breast cancer in general. Eight per cent are simultaneously bilateral and a further 20% metachronous.

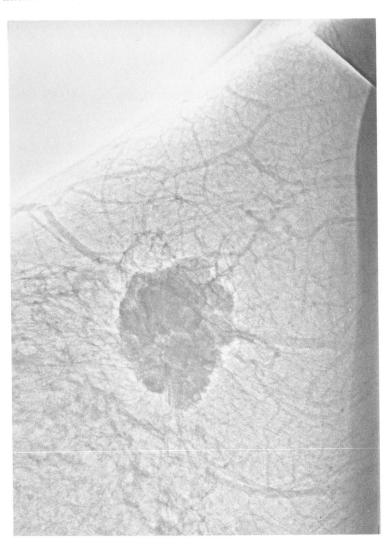

Fig. 6.10 A carcinoma with a mainly nodular outline and some spiculations.

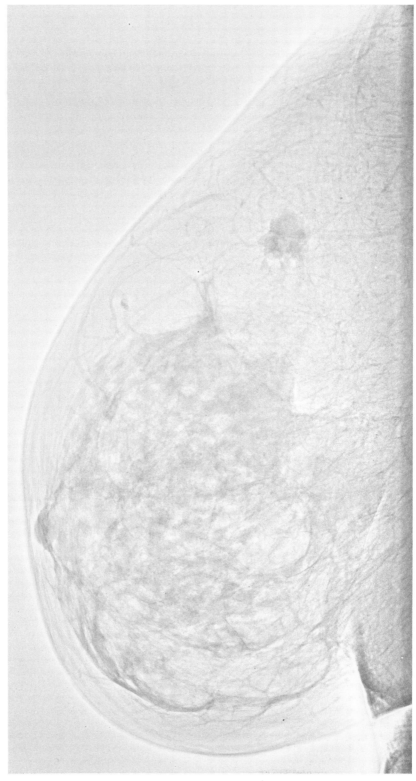

Fig. 6.11   A small nodular carcinoma lies in the fat above the breast parenchyma in a patient aged 60. It is not too unusual to see tumours in this site, they presumably arise in residual parenchyma left behind as the breast atrophies.

Discrete masses

In 85% of breast tumours the boundary of the area of increased density is well enough defined to be recognized as a discrete mass. This is most often spiculated or irregularly nodular but may be round or lobulated. Spiculation is a very strong indicator of malignancy, 98% of such masses which come to biopsy are malignant (Figs 6.1–6.3). The tumour contains a considerable amount of fibrous tissue and there may be permeation of tumour cells amongst the fibrous strands as well as along adjacent ducts. These tumours fulfill Lebourgne's sign, that on palpation the tumour appears much larger than on the mammogram.

The irregular nodularity of some carcinoma masses is due to the coalescence of separate nodules of intraduct carcinoma (Figs 6.10 and 6.11). Occasionally, nodules may be seen remote from the main mass due to spread along the periductal lymphatics. Less than 5% of carcinomas have sharply marginated, round or lobulated outlines. These include

Fig. 6.12   A medullary carcinoma showing very well-defined smooth margins with no evidence of infiltration into the surrounding tissue.

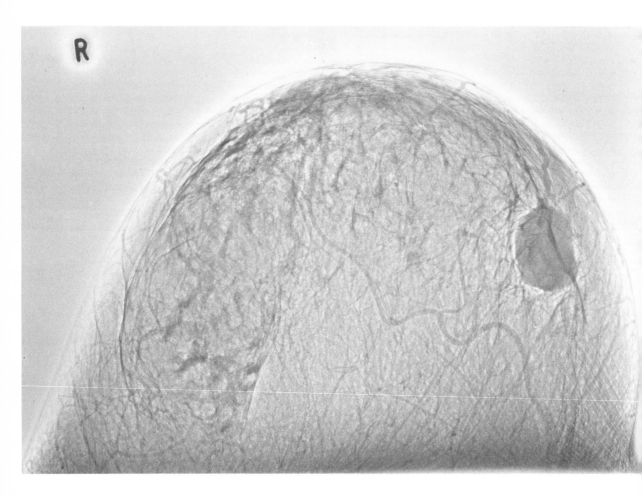

Fig. 6.13 A well-defined lobulated mucoid carcinoma.

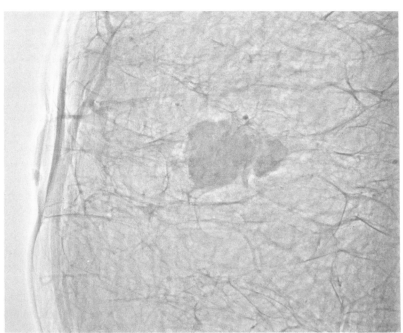

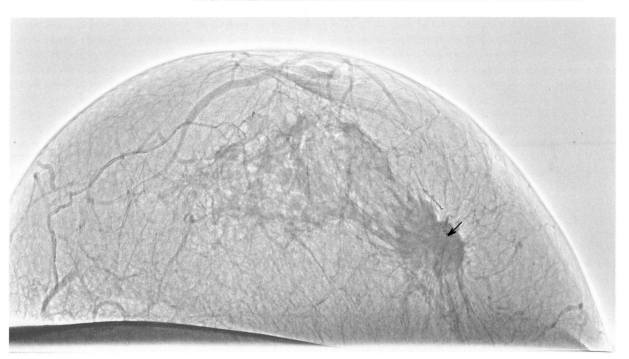

Fig. 6.14 A positive mode cranio-caudad view shows an infiltrating ductal carcinoma which has a partly rounded and partly spiculated outline. There is adjacent arterial calcification (arrow).

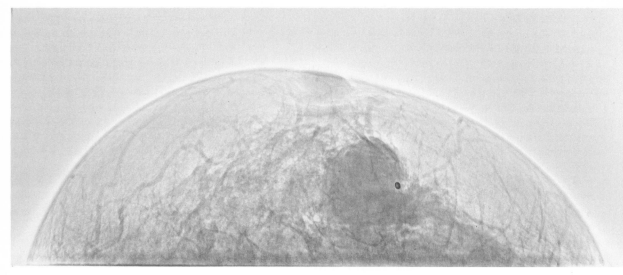

Fig. 6.15   Although this carcinoma is well defined anteriorly and shows a more or less rounded outline, the posterior surface is poorly defined and irregular where there is infiltration into the surrounding tissue. The ring calcification is incidental.

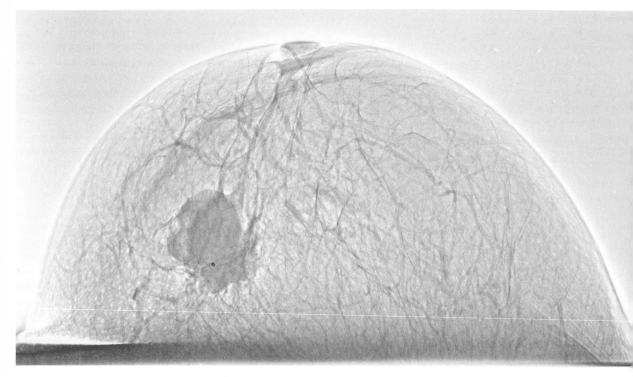

Fig. 6.16   A similar carcinoma to Fig. 6.7 showing a predominantly rounded mass but with tumour extending into the surrounding breast tissue.

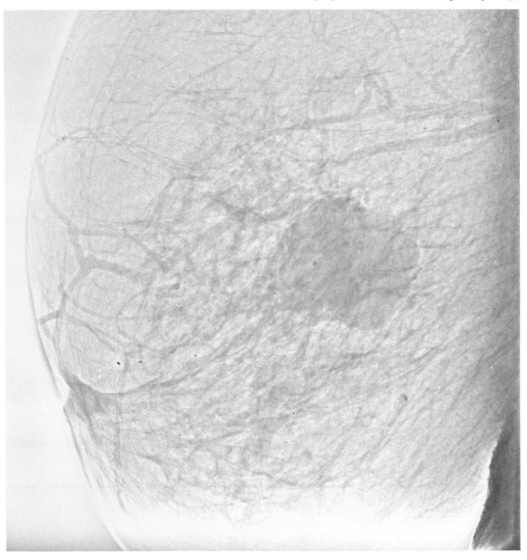

Fig. 6.17   Mucoid carcinoma with a predominantly well-defined lobulated margin but less clearly identifiable anteriorly where it is extending along ducts toward the inverted nipple.

medullary, mucoid and intracystic papillary tumours but also occasionally the more aggressive infiltrating ductal lesions (Figs 6.12 and 6.13). Sharply defined, rounded masses are much more commonly benign so that there is a danger of issuing a false negative report. The periphery of these lesions often shows some slight irregularity or spiculation which indicates infiltration of the tumour into the surrounding tissue (Figs 6.14–6.17). Nevertheless, many of these lesions will be smooth in their entire outline

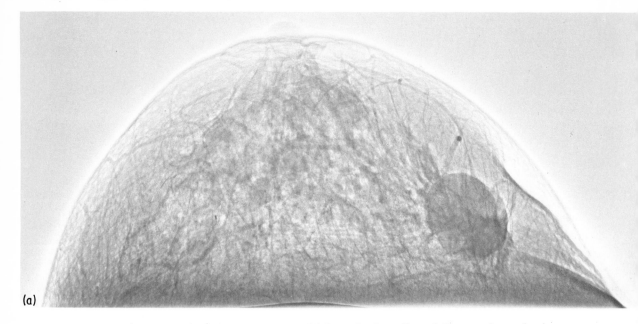

(a)

Fig. 6.18 (a) A rounded mass is associated with skin retraction and with spiculation adjacent to its anterior border. This is a cyst obscuring a carcinoma. (b) Following aspiration of the cyst the carcinoma is revealed in the upper part of the breast (arrow).

even on multiple projections. Even failure to change in size over two or three years should not be taken as evidence of benignity as some breast carcinomas have a very low doubling rate as Heuser, Spratt and Polk, 1979, have shown. If the patient is in the high tumour-risk age group, that is over the age of 40, it is best to indicate that whilst the lesion is most likely benign, cancer cannot be excluded and biopsy or cytology should be obtained.

Payne and Jackson, 1980, found that intracystic papillary tumours account for only 0.5% of all breast cancers (Fig. 6.19). They characteristically occur after the menopause when simple cysts are uncommon. In half of my own cases tumour has been demonstrated infiltrating through the wall of the cyst into the adjacent tissue (Fig. 6.20). However, there may be no mammographic signs to distinguish these lesions from simple cysts. Characteristically these tumours are slow growing and late to metastasize. Benign intracystic papillary tumours are 3 times as common as intracystic carcinomas. After the menopause cysts should be aspirated and further clinical and mammographic examinations undertaken to rule out a residual mass. Cysts containing tumour refill very readily so that the patient should be reviewed after six weeks. Blood in the cyst fluid is a very suspicious sign. When these features are present pneumocystography may be helpful in showing irregularity of the cyst wall due to tumour, but, many workers would recommend biopsy whatever the cystogram showed.

Medullary carcinomas are nearly always very sharply outlined and may be round, ovoid or lobulated (Fig. 6.12). They never calcify. Mucoid carcinomas may present either as an ill-defined area of increased density or as a well-defined mass and about half contain some calcification (Figs 6.13

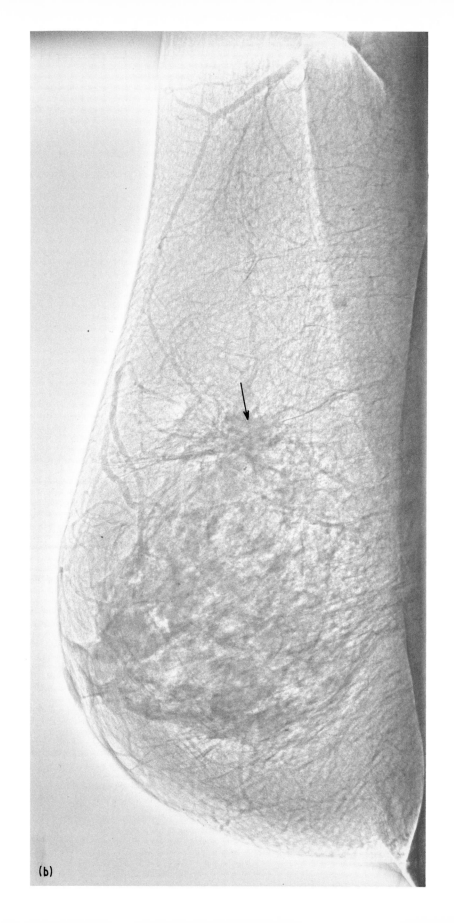

(b)

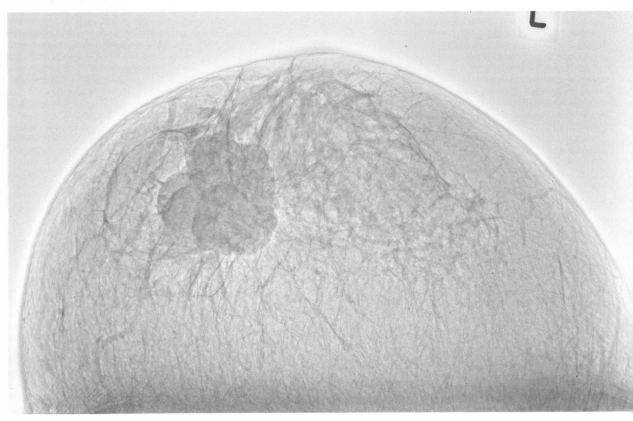

Fig. 6.19   A lobulated cystic mass giving no clue to the papillary carcinoma within.

and 6.17). Very rarely lace-like calcification is the only sign of a mucoid tumour (Fig. 6.21).

Breast tumours are popularly thought of as enlarging equally in all directions but in fact there is often a predominant enlargement of tumour in the direction of the ducts towards the nipple (Fig. 6.22). One or more dilated ducts may be demonstrated extending from tumour to nipple and rarely a solitary enlarged duct is the only sign of tumour. Ducts of exactly similar appearance may be seen due to obstruction by papilloma, inspissated secretions or duct ectasia. Asymmetric ductal enlargement is an important sign which may lead to the detection of a deep tumour mass.

Disturbed architecture

Uncommonly, a tumour will be recognized by the distortion of surrounding structures rather than as a localized increase in density (Fig. 6.23). As tumours enlarge they displace the normal ligaments of Astley-Cooper or engulf them so that they can no longer be seen (the silhouette sign). These are unusual signs which in a recent review (Parsons, 1981) the author found

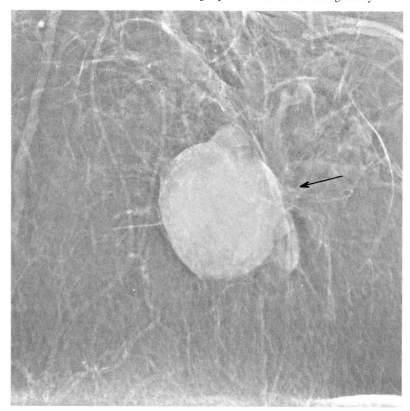

Fig. 6.20 Negative mode xerogram of a papillary intracystic carcinoma invading the adjacent tissue (arrow).

in only 3 of 607 cancers. Exactly similar appearances may be seen in sclerosing adenosis and in scarring after surgery.

Calcification

The detection of calcification is extremely important to the diagnosis of malignant breast lesions. There is no single feature of the calcific particles which is characteristic of malignancy. Rather, the radiologist must look for a combination of features which together imply malignancy. The features which must be assessed are:

1. Association of calcification with a mass.
2. Distribution
    (a) in groups.
    (b) along ducts.
3. Size.
4. Shape.
5. Concommitant Paget's disease.

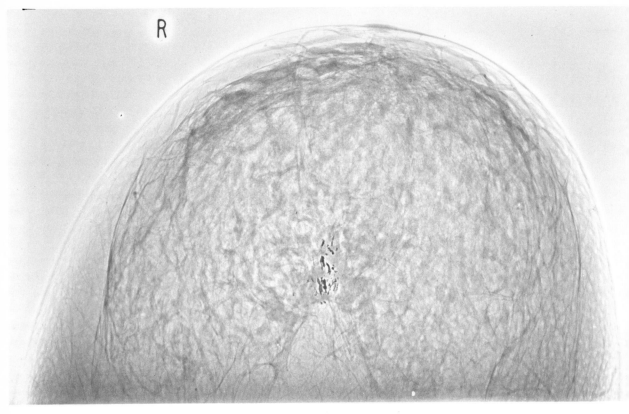

Fig. 6.21   Large lace-like calcifications in a mucoid carcinoma.

Calcification associated with a malignant mass may lie wholly within the mass or may, in addition, extend into the surrounding tissue usually following the course of a duct towards the nipple (Figs 6.25–6.29). Many benign masses also contain calcification and difficulty in interpretation will most commonly arise with sclerosing adenosis, papillomatosis and fat necrosis. The appearance of the calcification in these conditions may be so like those of cancer that some false positive reports are inevitable. Ninety per cent of masses containing calcification and requiring biopsy, that is excluding obvious degenerated fibroadenomas or cysts with mural calcification, are found to be malignant. An even higher proportion are malignant if the mass is spiculated or nodular.

The distribution of calcifications is a most important feature. Localized grouping of calcifications is suspicious whether associated with a mass or not (Figs 6.31 and 6.32). Grouping is only difficult to recognize when there are, in addition, multiple diffuse calcifications due to benign mammary dysplasia. When this occurs a particularly diligent search must be made for any area in which the character of the calcifications is different.

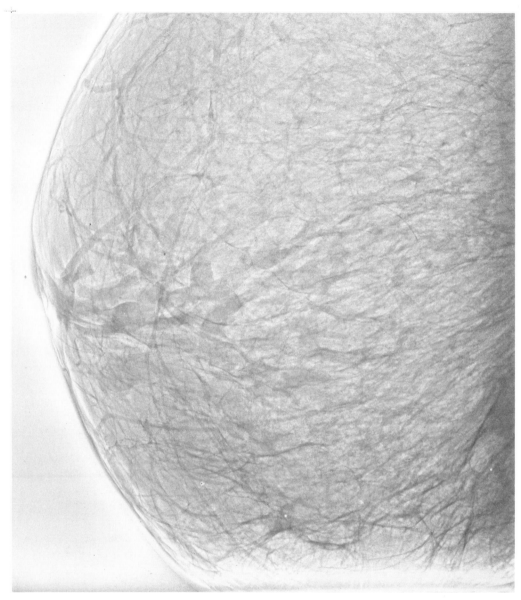

Fig. 6.22   Enlargement of the ducts immediately deep to the nipple due to tumour permeation without infiltration into the adjacent breast parenchyma.

Calcification in benign mammary dysplasia is usually fairly symmetrical. Grouped calcifications may also be seen in several benign conditions particularly sclerosing adenosis, papillomatosis, fat necrosis or in the wall of a cyst.

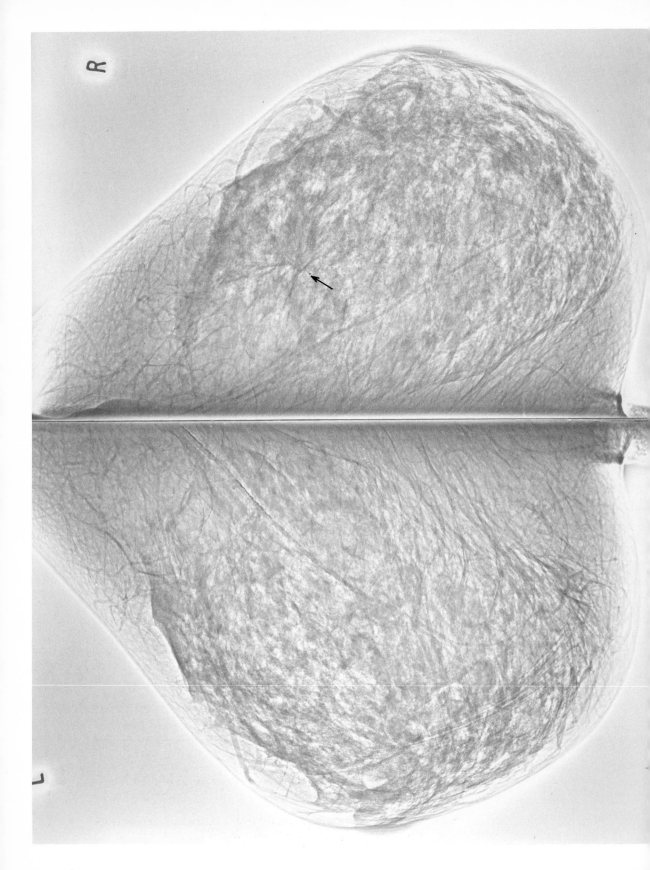

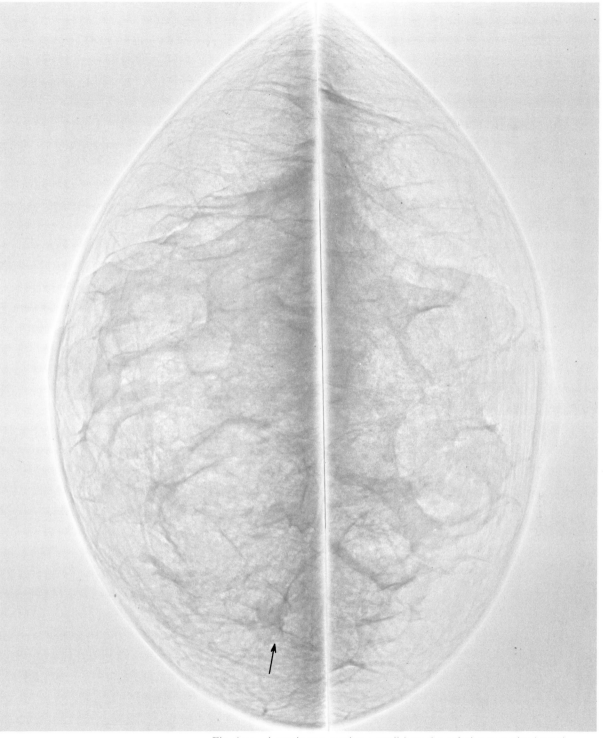

Fig. 6.24 A carcinoma causing a small irregular soft tissue opacity (arrow). Lesions of this type will only be detected by comparing similar areas of the two breasts.

◀ Fig. 6.23 Disturbed architecture due to carcinoma in the upper part of the right breast (arrow). The tumour has caused spiculations due to fibrosis without forming a definable mass.

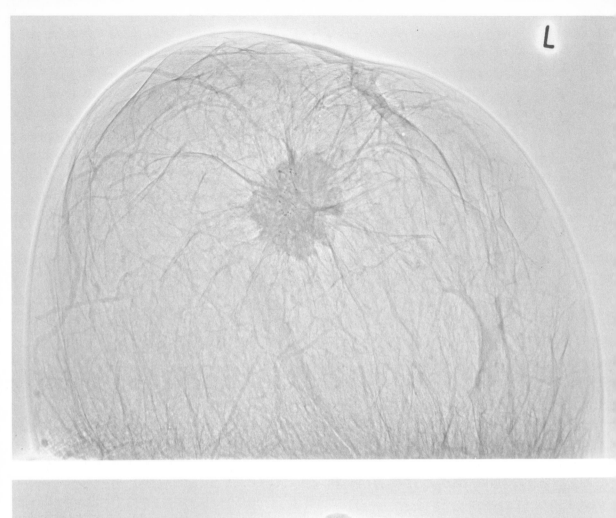

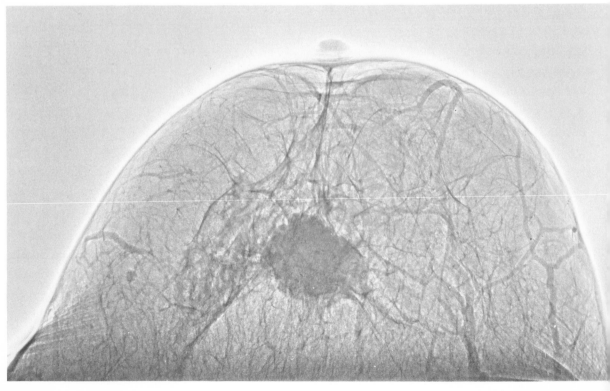

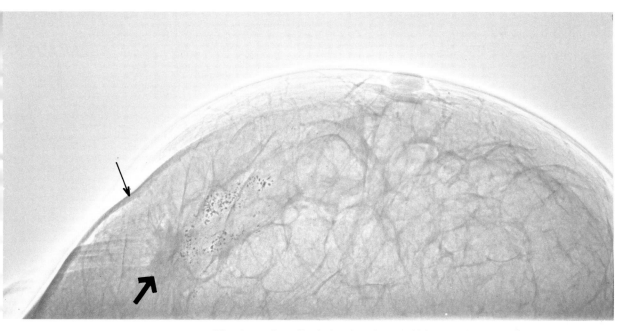

Fig. 6.27 A small spiculated carcinoma (thick arrow) is causing skin retraction (thin arrow) and there are round and regular calcifications extending toward the nipple.

Fig. 6.25 (*Upper*) A spiculated carcinoma containing small round calcifications.

Fig. 6.26 (*Lower*) A nodular carcinoma containing multiple very fine microcalcifications.

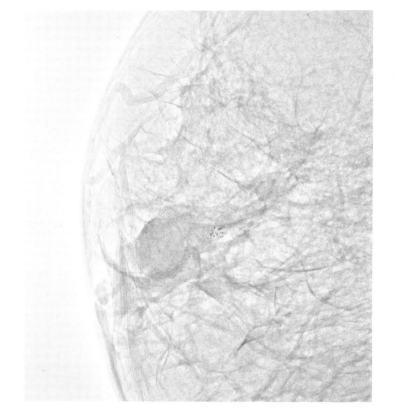

Fig. 6.28 An infiltrating carcinoma containing a small group of calcifications and a well-defined soft tissue component which contains mucin.

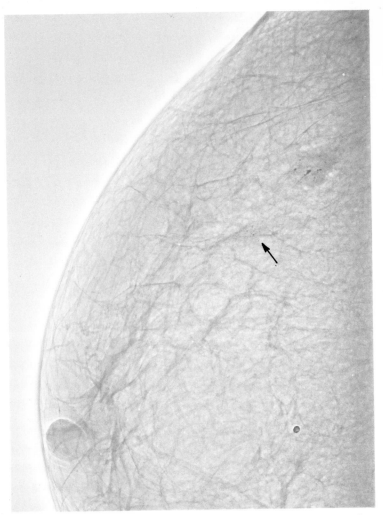

Fig. 6.29   A small tumour mass contains multiple calcifications with a further group of very fine calcifications (arrow) lying near to the nipple.

Intraduct carcinoma particularly of the comedo variety may be evident solely as calcification along the duct system (Figs 6.33–6.35). This type of tumour may occupy a large proportion of the breast and still remain impalpable. Occasionally, Paget's disease of the nipple is the only clinical sign to indicate the presence of such an underlying tumour.

A variety of sizes and shapes of calcification are found together in carcinomas. No calcification is too small to represent malignancy and the majority are less than 0.5 mm in diameter. Occasionally, some particles 2–3 mm in diameter will be seen and rarely all the calcifications are of this size. In benign mammary dysplasia the calcifications are also most commonly less than 0.5 mm in diameter so that size is not a good indicator of malignancy.

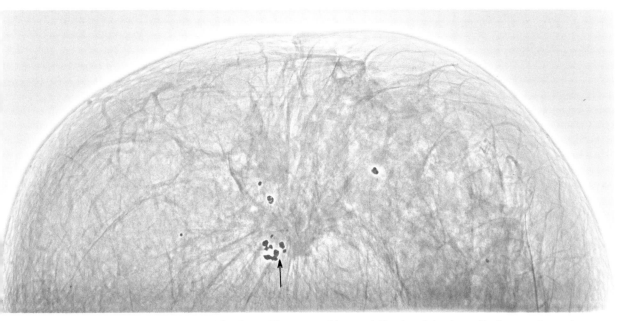

Fig. 6.30 The group of large calcifications lying immediately posterior to the spiculated carcinoma are in an incidental degenerated fibroadenoma.

The calcium particles are most commonly smooth and round (Figs 6.25 and 6.26) and these have been shown to occur within viable tumour (Millis *et al.*, 1976). This type of calcification can be identical to that found in benign mammary dysplasia. Within necrotic tumour the calcifications are often small and irregular in outline. Linear calcifications, usually very slim but occasionally as broad as 2 mm and extending up to 4–5 mm in length, are usually good evidence of malignancy when confined to a small area or segment of the breast (Fig. 6.36). The linear calcifications lie along the course of the ducts so that they spread along a radius towards the nipple (Fig. 6.37). The ductal location may be emphasized by branching and this may be well enough developed to form a lace-like pattern. This branched calcification must be differentiated from that seen in secretory disease. In this benign condition linear calcifications, sometimes branching, are commonly seen. They are nearly always wider than those seen in malignancy, being 2 mm or more in diameter and commonly 1 cm in length. Their tubular nature is often evident due to a lucent centre so that when seen end on they appear as rings. Secretory disease is nearly always bilateral and often affects the whole breast so that in practice differentiation of the two conditions is usually straightforward.

The shape of calcifications is helpful in balancing a mammographic opinion. Angular and linear calcifications are 4 times as common in cancers which contain calcification than in those benign mammary dysplasias which contain calcification. Round calcifications are equally common in the two conditions.

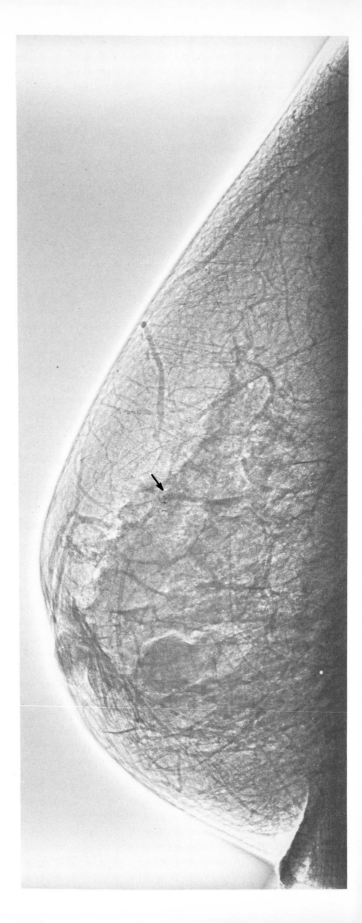

Fig. 6.31   A very small group of
microcalcifications (arrow) mark the
site of lobular *in situ* carcinoma. A cyst
is present in the lower part of the
breast.

Fig. 6.32 A group of quite large calcifications due to an infiltrating intraduct carcinoma.

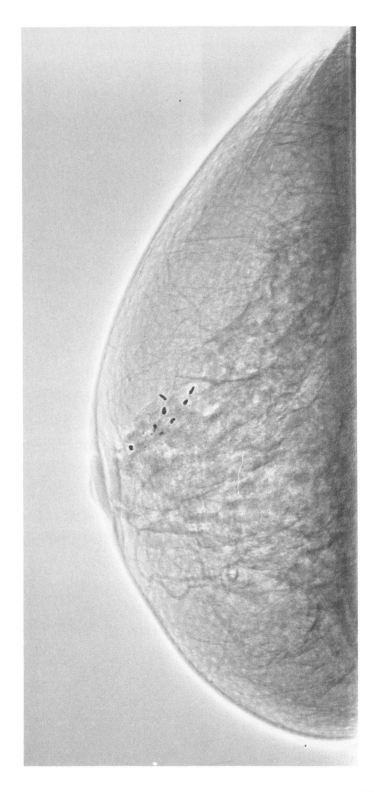

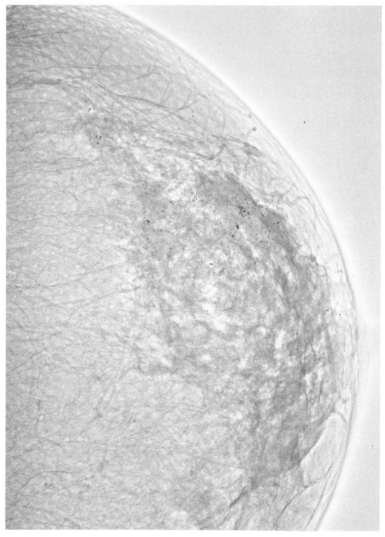

Fig. 6.33 Fairly diffuse fine calcification due to the comedo-type of intraduct carcinoma.

Fig. 6.34 An impalpable comedo carcinoma occupying the upper half of the breast. ▶

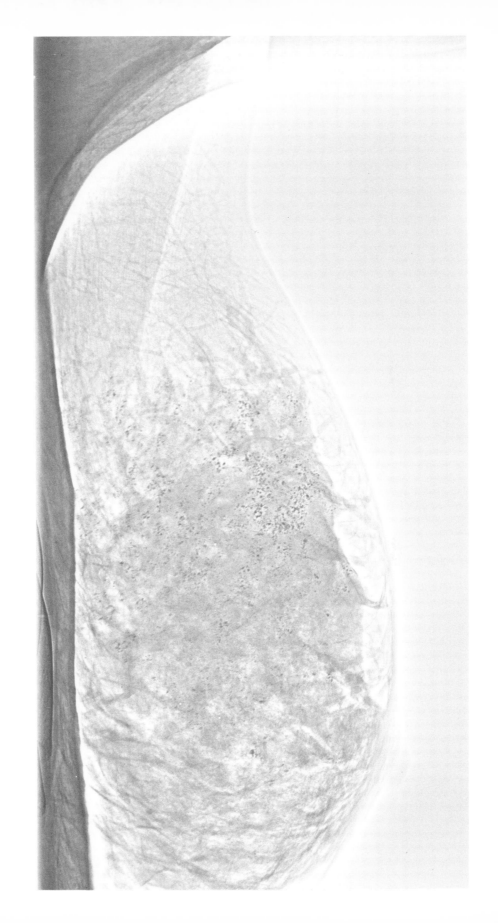

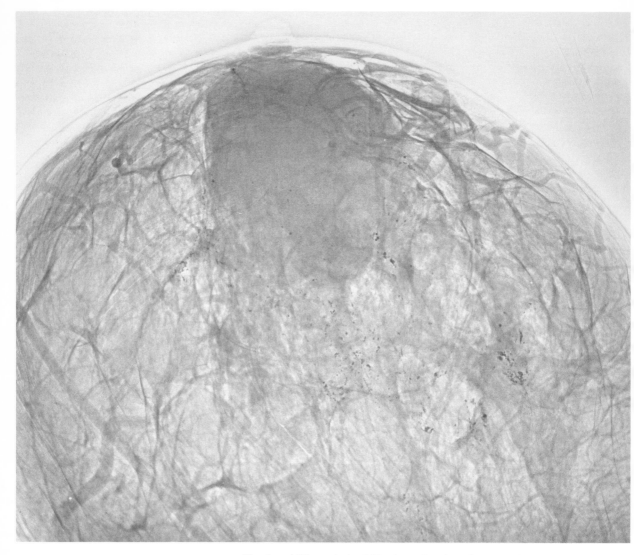

Fig. 6.35   The typical calcifications of an intraduct comedo carcinoma occupy a considerable area of the breast with a large incidental cyst immediately deep to the nipple.

The number of calcifications on its own is not a useful guide to the malignancy of a lesion. Quite frequently, obviously malignant masses will contain only one small round calcification. Occasionally, just 2 or 3 calcifications grouped together with no evidence of a mass will be the sole evidence of a tumour, particularly lobular-*in situ*. In screening projects small groups of calcification have been the only means of detecting up to

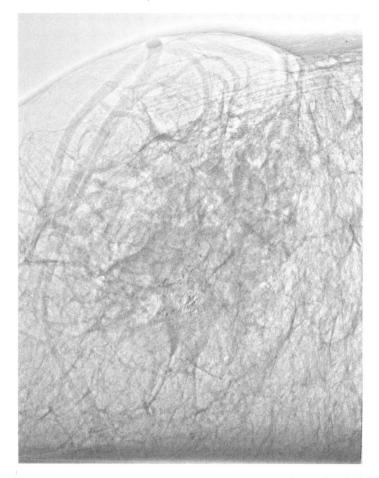

Fig. 6.36   Linear and branching calcifications typical of carcinoma lie within an area of increased density.

50% of the clinically occult tumours. Although, 2 or 3 calcifications grouped together may indicate a malignant lesion the radiologist should issue a balanced report since exactly similar findings are more common in benign disease. There is no value in the policy of following the patient with a further mammogram after a few months to show if the number of calcifications increases or if a mass develops to give more certainty of malignancy. If the patient has cancer she should be diagnosed at the time of presentation. If the mammographic diagnosis cannot be certain, needle aspiration of the suspicious area should be carried out for cytology. If there is still doubt then biopsy should be advised. It is in this situation that needle localization prior to biopsy and specimen radiography to confirm excision are most helpful.

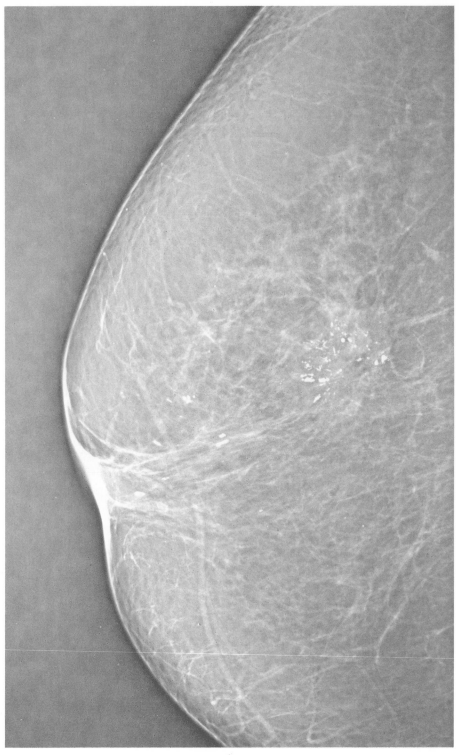

Fig. 6.37 A negative mode lateral view of a carcinoma containing round and linear calcifications, some of which are branching. Further calcifications extend from the tumour mass along ducts towards the nipple.

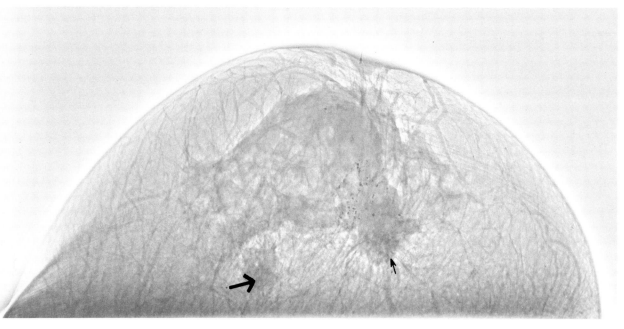

Fig. 6.38 Multifocal carcinoma. The larger tumour (small arrow) is associated with calcifications extending toward the nipple. The smaller tumour (large arrow) is evident only as a spiculated soft tissue mass.

INDIRECT EVIDENCE OF MALIGNANCY

Skin changes

Comparison of the radiological features of benign and malignant breast lesions shows that excluding surgery skin changes are almost completely confined to the cancer group. In my own study (Parsons, 1981) 177 cancers showed skin abnormalities amongst a total group of 613, whilst only 7 patients out of 539 with benign disease had similar changes. A high reliance can be placed on these features in supporting the diagnosis of cancer.

Important skin changes may be overlooked when there are more obvious abnormalities within the breast itself. This can be avoided if the radiologist develops the habit of always examining the skin first, comparing each area of one breast with the other.

Skin thickening may occur diffusely throughout the breast or may be localized to a smaller area overlying a superficial tumour (Fig. 6.39). Localized skin thickening may be caused by direct extension of tumour into the skin or by obstruction of the subdermal lymphatics causing cutaneous oedema (Fig. 6.40). This may occur with any infiltrating carcinoma but is most florid in the inflammatory tumours (Fig. 6.7).

Fig. 6.39 The most obvious skin change due to tumour, direct invasion.

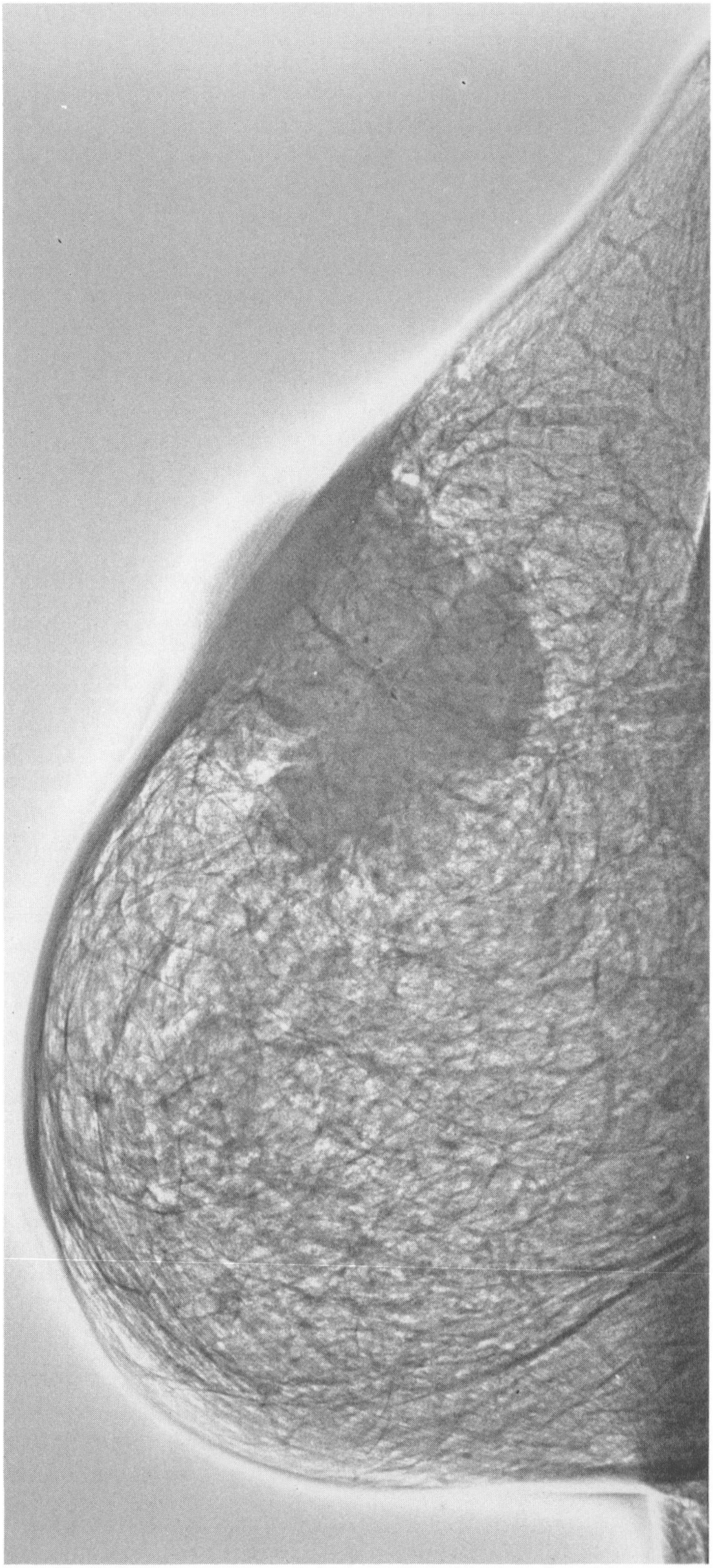

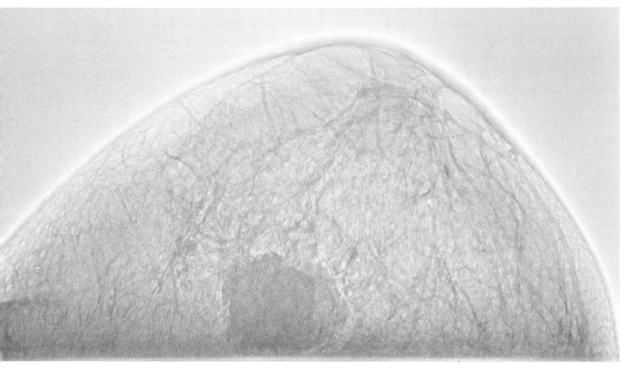

Fig. 6.40   Peri-areolar oedema associated with a deep carcinoma.

Intraduct carcinoma involving the nipple frequently spreads directly into the skin of the areola and can be recognized on the mammogram as thickening. This appearance is identical to that due to Paget's disease. Diffuse skin thickening may also be caused by direct skin infiltration or by obstruction to the axillary lymph nodes by metastases (Fig. 6.41). This may be seen in lymphomas involving the axilla whether the breast parenchyma is involved or not. Obstruction to the axillary lymphatics or vein as a result of previous surgery may also cause diffuse cutaneous oedema.

Diffuse skin thickening and a generalized increase in breast density particularly of the reticular fibres which pass through the subcutaneous fat is seen commonly after radiotherapy. The change begins after the first 4 or 5 weeks of treatment, remains very marked for several months and often improves over the course of the next year.

A very interesting group of patients with skin thickening are those with an advanced tumour in the medial part of the breast which spreads across the midline to cause skin thickening in the medial part of the opposite breast. This is due to direct skin infiltration and subdermal lymphatic permeation.

Skin or nipple retraction is seen three or four times more frequently

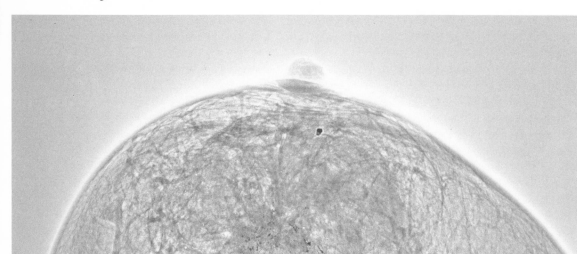

Fig. 6.41   A large central spiculated carcinoma with an associated involved intramammary lymph node (arrow). There is skin thickening laterally.

than skin thickening (Figs 6.42 and 6.43). Scirrhous carcinomas provoke fibrosis in the surrounding tissue and when they lie superficially, contraction of the fibrous tissues may cause first of all flattening of the normal convex breast outline and eventually localized puckering (Fig. 6.44). This may be evident on only one view and only when the affected area of skin is shown in profile. The radiographer may be the first to notice skin retraction since it may become evident only on compressing the breast. The involved skin may be greater in density than the rest of the skin of that breast or a similar area in the opposite breast. The same process which causes skin dimpling may lead to nipple retraction. This is particularly common since such a high proportion of breast cancer is due to infiltrating ductal tumours which spread forward to the nipple. This is a common clinical abnormality and whilst it should always alert the radiologist to the possibility of an underlying tumour this is by no means always the case. Nipple retraction may occur without any radiologically apparent underlying abnormality and is very common in secretory disease when there is usually good clinical and mammographic evidence of the cause.

Increased vascularity

Asymmetry in the diameter of mammary blood vessels and the disparity in

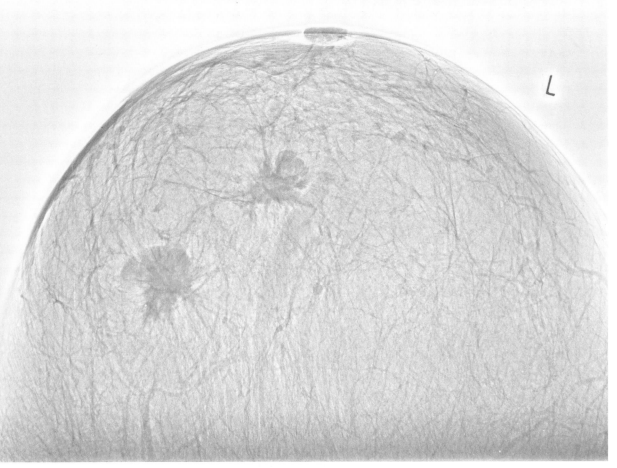

Fig. 6.42   Multiple spiculated carcinomas with thickening and slight retraction of the adjacent skin.

their number between the two sides is occasionally seen in completely normal patients and accompanying benign disease. It has been suggested that a blood vessel diameter of 1.5 times that in a similar position of the opposite breast was abnormal. Precise measurement of that type is not practical since it varies with positioning and compression. In 40 out of 613 cancers, I have found an obvious increase in vascularity to the affected area. Only 6 out of 539 benign abnormalities showed a similar change. This sign is of very little value on its own but it should be given considerable weight when it accompanies other suspicious features. Asymmetric increase in vascularity is most often found in the most rapidly growing carcinomas and sarcomas.

When comparing the vascularity of serial mammograms it is important to recognize the change which occurs throughout the menstrual cycle. A

Fig. 6.43 A carcinoma directly invading the skin and causing retraction associated with extension along ducts toward the nipple.

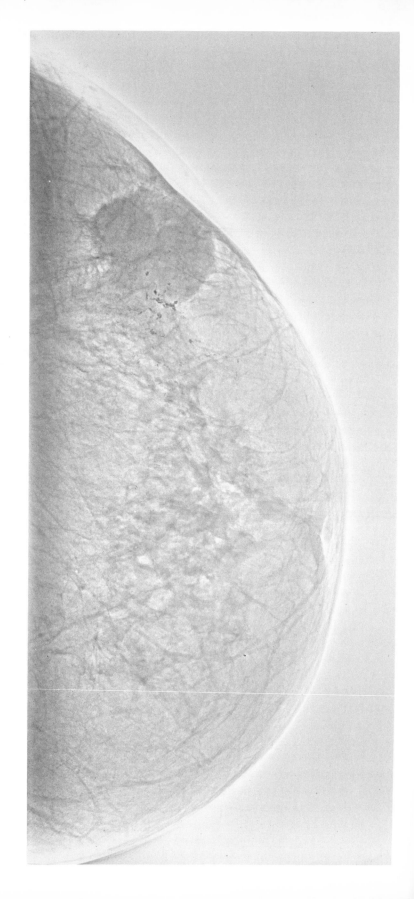

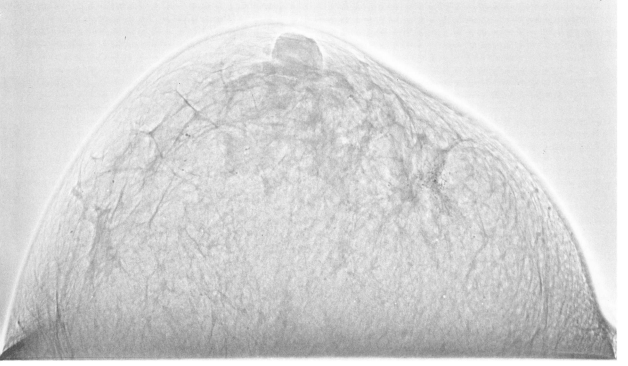

Fig. 6.44 A small superficial carcinoma containing multiple
microcalcifications is causing skin flattening, the first step in skin retraction.

bilateral increase in vascularity can occur premenstrually usually in
patients with mastalgia and usually accompanied by generalized blurring
of detail due to oedema.

Axillary lymph node assessment

To recognize the features of lymph node metastases one has to be familiar
with normal appearance (Fig. 5.13). Most nodes are oval in shape with a
longitudinal dimension of less than 2 cm and a transverse diameter of up
to 1 cm. Smaller completely round nodes with a diameter of less than 1 cm
are frequently seen and may be numerous. Lucent areas due to fat
replacement are common in the axillary lymph nodes (Fig. 6.45).

Metastases cause enlargement compared with nodes in the same or the
other axilla and a change to a more spherical shape. In the presence of a
breast tumour nodes with a completely rounded outline and a diameter of
greater than 1 cm should be regarded as probably involved by metastases
(Figs 6.41, 6.45 and 6.47). Very rarely punctate calcifications are present
within lymph node deposits (Fig. 6.48).

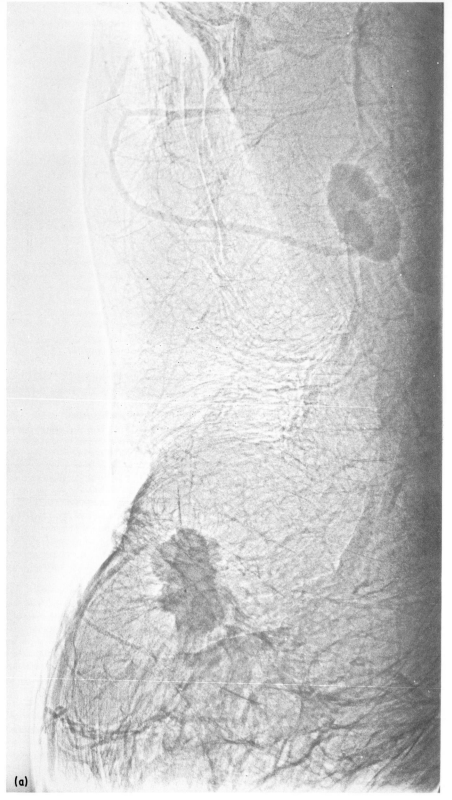

(a)

Fig. 6.45 (a) A carcinoma in the axillary tail with an adjacent involved lymph node in the lower part of the axilla. (b) Another carcinoma in the axillary tail. The lowest axillary lymph node shows fatty replacement. None of the nodes contained metastases at histology.

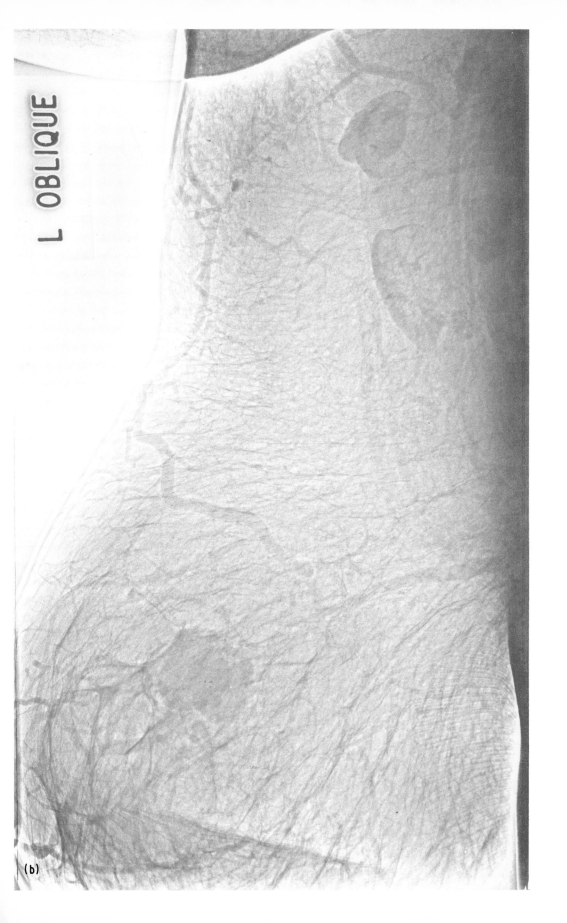

L OBLIQUE

(b)

L OBLIQUE

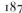

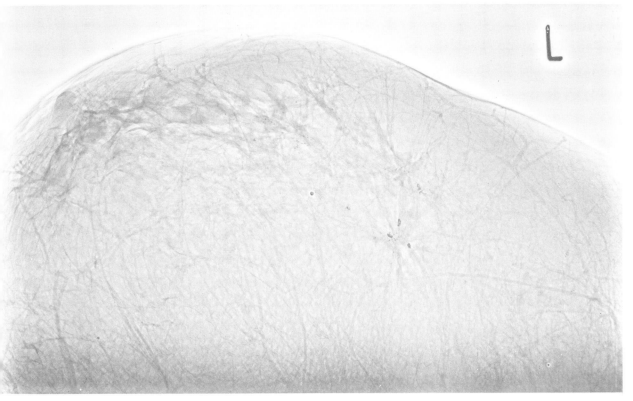

Fig. 6.47 Extended cranio-caudad view of a tumour in the lateral part of the breast with two involved lymph nodes completely replaced by tumour with invasion of the surrounding axillary fat.

Using these criteria a radiological assessment that lymph nodes are involved is usually proved to be correct by histology. That is about 85% of positive radiological reports are shown to be true positives. However, a negative assessment is of no value since about half of the cases so reported will be found to have lymph node metastases by histology. This is due to failure to show some nodes amongst the other axillary tissues and failure to show micrometastases in nodes of completely normal appearance, even in the rim of remaining lymphoid tissue in a node almost completely replaced by fat. There is some improvement in the accuracy of radiological assessment as the number of lymph nodes shown histologically to contain metastases increases.

PARENCHYMAL PATTERNS

◀ Fig. 6.46 Huge axillary lymph nodes due to lymphoma.

There has been interest in the mammographic appearance of the breast parenchyma for many years with attempts to determine if a particular

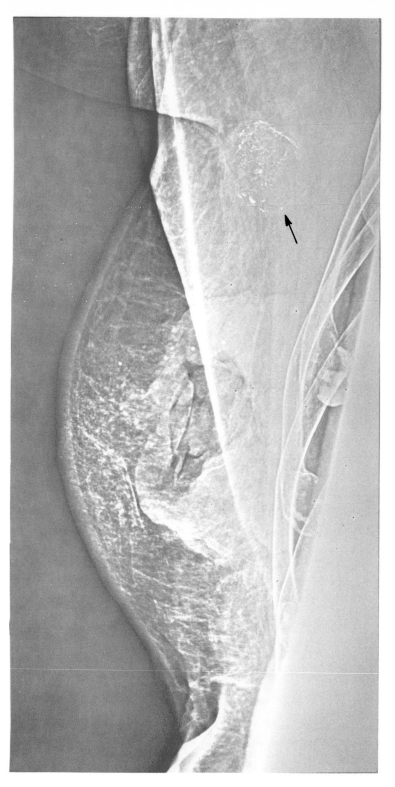

Fig. 6.48 A very advanced ulcerated carcinoma with calcification in a lymph node deposit (arrow).

pattern favours the development of breast cancer. In 1976 Wolfe published a study which claimed that it was possible to identify a high risk group in this way. He described 4 groups classified as follows:

N1. In which the parenchyma is composed primarily of fat with at most small areas of increased density due to dysplasia, but no identifiable ducts (Fig. 6.1).

P1. The parenchyma is mostly fat with prominent ducts in the anterior portion of the breast or occupying up to one quadrant but always less than one quarter of the volume of the breast.

P2. A prominent duct pattern occupies greater than one quarter, and frequently the whole of the breast (Fig. 6.2).

DY. Ill-defined areas of increased density are present which in the grossest cases may be confluent. The densities represent the fibrous element of benign mammary dysplasia (Fig. 5.1).

The ducts are recognized as linear and nodular densities extending away from the nipple. Histological and radiographic correlation of these appearances by Wellings and Wolfe (1978) has shown these densities to be due to periductal and perilobular fibrosis. The same pathological study found a step-wise increase in the frequency of atypical epithelial changes thought to be precancerous from N1 through P1 to a high incidence in P2 and DY categories.

Two groups of women were included in Wolfe's (1976a) original report. All had an initial normal mammogram and were followed for the subsequent development of breast cancer. In one group 85% of the cancers developed in 33% of the patients, that is, those with P2 and DY patterns. In the second group the same parenchymal patterns comprised 46.8% of the population and contained 95% of the cancers. Wolfe suggested that the stimulus to develop cancer also causes a prominent duct pattern and acts to prevent the normal regression of mammary dysplasia.

The hypothesis is important since limited screening resources could be used for those at greatest risk (P2 and DY) and patients at low risk (N1 and P1) could be spared the possibly harmful effects of unnecessary radiation.

Numerous reports have followed this important work. Virtually no author has denied the presence of the parenchymal pattern groups and the majority have found cancers predominantly in the P2 and DY groups. There have been some reports of other findings. Enster *et al.*, 1980, found cancer patients and controls similarly distributed across the parenchymal types, the majority in each group being P2 and DY. Egan and MacSweeney, 1979, found a majority of their prevalent tumours were accompanied by N1 and P1 patterns but a majority of their incident tumours were in the P2 and DY groups. They concluded that no mammographic pattern can reveal which women have a significantly higher risk of developing cancer. They suggested that there was a correlation with a failure to detect a lesion at the patient's first mammography if it was obscured by dense, dysplastic tissue and this accounted for the subsequent high rate of cancer development in the DY group.

One would expect some relationship to be apparent between parenchymal patterns and other recognized risk factors such as family history, previous breast cancer and parity if the patterns were reliable risk predictors. Wolfe (1976b) was not able to find any such relationship but Enster *et al.* (1980) found nulliparous women and women with a family history of breast cancer were most likely to fall into the P2 and DY categories. Similarly, Gravelle *et al* (1980) has reported a significantly higher proportion of P2 and DY patterns amongst the nulliparous and women with a late first pregnancy and a decrease in the proportions of those patterns in patients taking steroid contraceptives.

In a retrospective comparison of cancer patients and women found to be disease free attending the Early Diagnostic Unit of my institution a significantly greater proportion of the cancer group did have a P2 parenchymal pattern, 37.3% compared with 14.7% in the controls (Fig. 6.49). There was a lesser increase in the DY category, 33.7% of the cancer group and 25.1% of the controls and far fewer cancer patients showed an N1 pattern, 21% compared with 54% of the controls. The greatest

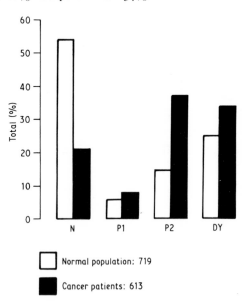

Fig. 6.49   Breast parenchymal patterns: comparision of normal and malignant populations.

☐ Normal population: 719

■ Cancer patients: 613

influence on the proportions of the various patterns was menopausal status. A decrease in the DY category occurs in postmenopausal women whether controls or cancer patients and the proportion with P2 increases (Figs 6.50 and 6.51). However, we have found no correlation with other risk factors such as parity, age at first pregnancy, breast feeding, contraceptive pills or family history. There was a strong correlation between the DY category and histological proof of benign mammary dysplasia.

At the time of writing the importance of parenchymal patterns has not been settled. Differences between centres presenting reports may be affected by the various mammographic techniques used and the better ability of some to demonstrate the ducts upon which assessment depends. The wisest use of the published information at present would seem to be for the radiologist to be even more cautious when interpreting suspicious but inconclusive mammograms when there is P2 or DY parenchymal pattern.

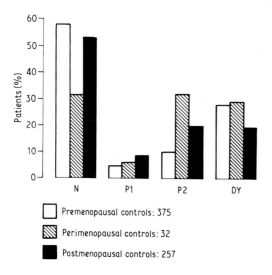

Fig. 6.50   Influence of hormonal status on breast parenchymal patterns of normal control group (719).

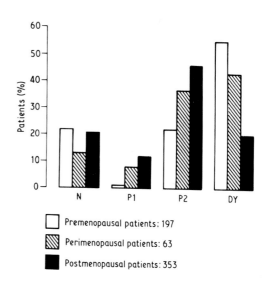

Fig. 6.51   Influence of hormonal status on breast parenchymal patterns in patients with cancer (613).

7 PRACTICAL DIAGNOSTIC PROCEDURES

C.A. Parsons and J.A. McKinna

PRE-OPERATIVE LOCALIZATION OF IMPALPABLE
BREAST LESIONS

One of the major benefits of modern mammographic technique is the demonstration of breast tumours before they have developed to the stage at which they are clinically apparent. These tumours are less often accompanied by lymph node metastases than those presenting symptomatically therefore becoming a prognostically favourable group. However, the demonstration of a mammographically suspicious but clinically occult lesion creates a considerable problem for the surgeon who is confronted with radiological evidence of an abnormality which he cannot feel in the patient and often cannot see at the time of biopsy. To avoid unnecessarily wide excision he may, quite reasonably, turn to the radiologist for assistance in accurately locating the lesion pre-operatively. Although this situation occurs most commonly in examination of apparently well women in screening projects, where approaching 50% of cancers are found by mammography alone, it will occur from time to time wherever a mammography service is provided. Various screening projects have reported that 20-40% of the radiologically suspicious lesions turn out to be cancers and they are impalpable due to small size or deep location.

The radiologist can help in two ways. Firstly, by locating the abnormality accurately prior to surgery and, secondly, by specimen radiography. Accurate localization simplifies and speeds the operation allowing a small volume of tissue to be removed so that there is diminished morbidity and a good cosmetic result. Patients accept the localization procedure very readily when these advantages are pointed out. A specimen radiograph should be made of the excised breast tissue to ensure that the radiologically abnormal area has been excised and to guide the pathologist to the most important area for histological study. The radiograph must be made before fixation of the specimen, which may leach out calcifications, and without unnecessary handling which may displace them. Although purely soft tissue abnormalities may be identifiable in the specimen the technique is most useful when calcifications are present.

Technique

Many techniques of localization of impalpable lesions have been tried and no single method has proved suitable for all abnormalities at all sites within the breast. There is something to be learned from most of the methods which have been shown to be unsatisfactory. The simplest procedure, used during the 1960s, required the radiologist to draw a diagram of the estimated position of the lesion after studying cranio-caudad and lateral mammograms. The surgeon planned his operation with the advantage of the drawing and found that in the supine patient relationships within the breast bear no resemblance to their position at mammography especially if compression has been used as is now the rule. The next method which had some advantage was to take small coned views (6 cm diameter) of the abnormality in the cranio-caudad and lateral projections marking the centring position on the patient's skin. These marks provide x and y co-ordinates of the lesion and the z co-ordinate (depth) can be estimated. This method has the same disadvantage of change in position when the patient is placed supine for surgery; nevertheless, if the surgeon is to carry out wide excision of the lesion these methods do offer some guidance. A similar principle was used by Frank and Rosenfeld (1973) who taped metallic numbers to the breast prior to standard mammographic projections and made marks on the skin at the numbers overlying the breast lesion.

All the other methods require introduction of a needle into the breast. Rosato *et al.* (1973) inserts multiple needles toward the expected site of the breast lesion as estimated from cranio-caudad and lateral films. He then repeats the mammographic exposures and removes all but the needle closest to the lesion. The discomfort caused to the patient by this method can, of course, be considerably reduced by more careful planning of a single needle insertion. A number of authors, amongst them Hornes and Arnolt (1976) and Simon *et al.* (1972), have advocated the injection of visible dye and radiographic contrast medium at the site of a lesion, as confirmed by mammogram with a needle in position, and injection of the dye along the tract as the needle is withdrawn. The technique requires biopsy to be carried out promptly since the dye will diffuse into the surrounding breast tissue particularly along ducts during the course of the next hour. In our experience on incising the breast the dye (Patent Blue Violet) stains all the surrounding tissue so that it is of very little help.

Amongst the complicated jigs and immobilisation devices which have been devised to assist in localization is one described by Mühlow (1974) is effective. The breast is radiographed whilst fixed in a plexi-glass compression device which has multiple perforations. A needle is passed through the hole under which the lesion is demonstrated and the procedure repeated in a plane at right angles to the first. The patient then proceeds to biopsy and the abnormality located where the needles cross.

Derived from these early procedures are two methods which can be recommended and which cover lesions at all sites within the breast. The

Fig. 7.1 (a) A preliminary cranio-caudad view shows a ring of platinum wire attached to the skin, marking the proposed site of needle entry, projected over grouped microcalcifications. (b) At the completion of the procedure a lateral view shows a hooked stylet has been advanced to the correct depth.

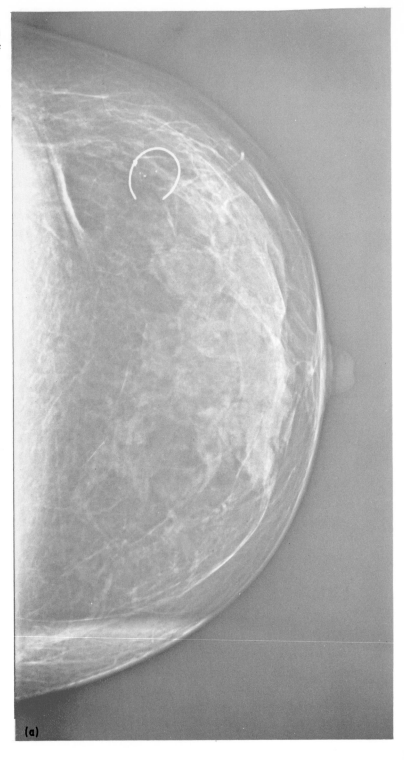

(a)

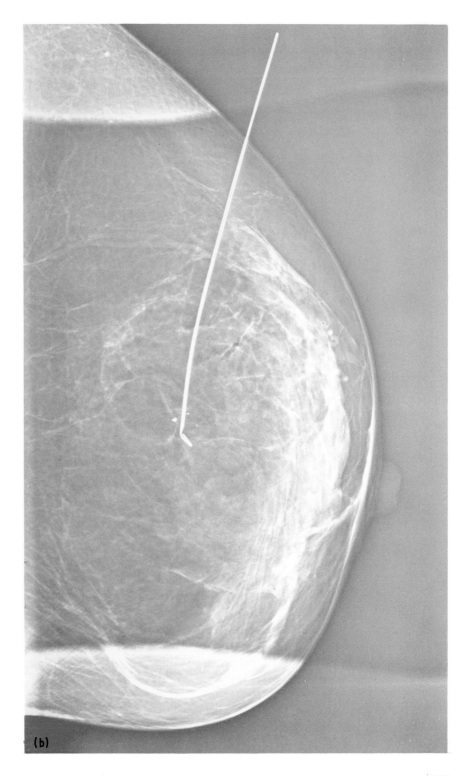

(b)

195

simplest, described by Peyster and Kalisher (1979), should be used whenever possible and certainly for all lesions in the upper half of the breast. On the patient's original cranio-caudad view a line is drawn perpendicular to the chest wall to pass through the nipple. A second line is drawn at right angles to the first to pass through the abnormality. Two measurements are made, one from the intersection of the lines to the nipple and, one from the intersection to the lesion. The patient is re-positioned for a further cranio-caudad view and the measurements are mapped out on the skin surface. A small ring of platinum wire is placed over the expected site of the lesion and a cranio-caudad projection made without compression (Fig. 7.1(a)). Usually the marker will overlie the lesion on the mammogram but if there is some slight error a corrected skin mark is made. The surrounding skin is cleaned and a small bleb of local anaesthetic is injected at the site of the skin mark. Only the skin need be anaesthetized since the underlying breast tissue is insensitive to the passage of a needle. The radiologist stands behind the patient who turns her head to the opposite side. A 20-gauge Frank needle with its hooked stylet withdrawn into the lumen of the needle is inserted to its full depth parallel to the chest wall. The needle is taped in position. A further cranio-caudad view is obtained to show that the needle transfixes the lesion and a lateral projection obtained from which the distance the needle has to be withdrawn for its tip to lie within the abnormality can be measured. When the needle has been withdrawn the appropriate amount, the hooked stylet is advanced (Fig. 7.1(b)). The stylets are extremely rigid so that if biopsy is not to take place within the next hour or two it is an advantage to cut the stylet off close to the skin and to cover the end with a plastic cap which is taped to the skin. An adaption of the method is to use 3–0 stainless steel suture, the end of which is bent into a hook in place of the stylet. This is malleable and can be bent along the skin surface. The surgeon cuts down onto the needle tip, through a circumareolar or cosmetic skin crease incision whenever possible, and obtains a small volume biopsy which is sent for specimen radiography. Even if the stylet tip is not precisely within the abnormality the radiologist is able to give very useful information concerning its precise relationship to the stylet tip.

The advantages of this method are that it is simple and accurate causing little discomfort to the patient who remains seated throughout the whole procedure. The direction in which the needle is advanced, perpendicular to the skin and parallel to the chest wall, avoids the possibility of pneumothorax which is present in some other methods.

Lesions in the lowermost part of the breast, particularly those lying very deep may not be reached by this method; in these circumstances the procedure described by Becker (1979) is useful. This method uses a radius drawn from the geometric centre of the breast on both cranio-caudad and lateral views through the nipple and through the abnormality (Fig. 7.2(a) and (b)). The distance on each film from the mid-point of the nipple to the point at which the radius through the breast lesion strikes the skin is

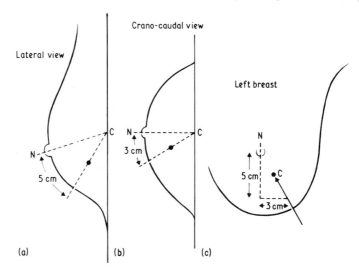

Fig. 7.2   Radii from the geometric centre of the breast (C) are drawn through the nipple and through the lesion on the lateral (a) and cranio-caudad (b) views. The distance on the skin between the exit points of these radii is measured. (c) A needle is advanced towards the geometric centre of the breast through a point determined by the skin measurements.

measured and transposed onto the patient's breast. Perpendiculars are drawn from the end of these lines and where they cross corresponds to the site of entry of the localizing needle. The Frank needle and stylet are inserted towards the estimated geometric centre of the breast to a depth estimated from the preliminary cranio-caudad and lateral views (Fig. 7.2(c)). Check mammograms in both planes are obtained and the needle tip adjusted for depth if necessary. If the needle tip is not within 1 cm of the lesion then a further needle can be inserted using the first as a guide. This method is also simple and accurate with a minimum of discomfort to the patient but requires practise at estimating the geometric centre of the breast.

Whenever a radiologist demonstrates an impalpable breast abnormality which is suspicious in appearance he has a responsibility to his surgical colleagues to aid in the localization of the abnormality at operation. The procedures described are simple and accurate and greatly facilitate the technique of biopsy.

DUCTOGRAPHY

Examination of the breasts by injection of radiographic contrast medium into a duct orifice on the nipple can provide useful information in the investigation of discharge from a single duct. This is particularly important when the discharge is serous or bloodstained. The investigation then becomes a useful preliminary to surgical exploration of the breast and the affected duct. It would be emphasized that the procedure is only one part of the investigation of such a discharge; it will follow physical examination, cytology of the secretion and conventional mammography.

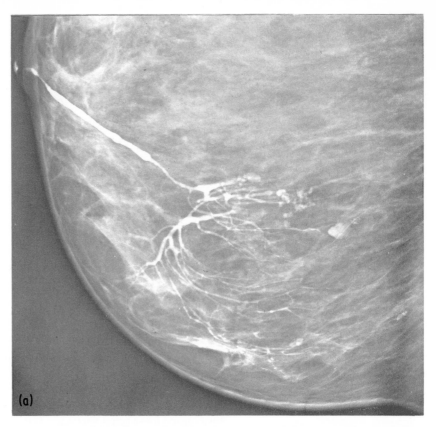

(a)

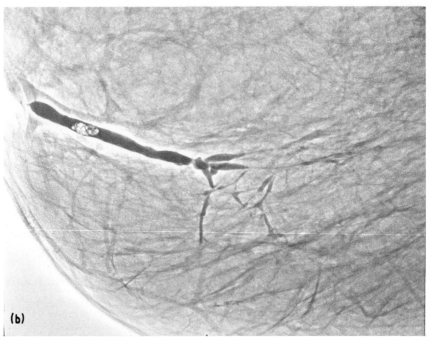

(b)

In many cases, it would precede and be complementary to surgical exploration and biopsy.

A bloody or serous discharge is usually associated with intraduct papilloma, less commonly with intraduct papillomatosis, which is often a premalignant condition, and, as patient age rises, the possibility of carcinoma increases (Funderburk and Syphax, 1969; Seltzer *et al.*, 1970). The demonstration of blood in a spontaneous nipple discharge is most easily achieved by the application of a diagnostic strip sensitive to blood. 'Haemastix' (Ames) diagnostic stick for the detection of blood in urine is suitable. The sensitive tip of the stick should be moistened with water immediately prior to its application to the discharge. This is a reliable and sensitive method of detecting blood, but, the cytological examination of the fluid is important as the cytologist will be observing the epithelial cells in the smear rather than merely erythrocytes.

Spontaneous discharge of fluid which is not bloodstained but which may vary in colour from white or grey to brown or green and which makes its appearance at several duct orifices in one or both breasts is almost always associated with benign mammary dysplasia in which there is a cystic component communicating with the major duct system of the breast. Creamy discharge may be a feature of duct ectasia. In such cases, contrast mammography can be time consuming and does not produce a useful yield of serious disease.

Technique

Early descriptions of intraductal injections come from Hicken (1937) and his colleagues (Hicken *et al.*, 1938) using thorotrast as the contrast medium. Later studies have reported the injection of ultra-fluid lipiodol or 50% sodium diatrizoate through fine, blunt needles (Bjorn-Hansen, 1965; Funderburk *et al.*, 1964; Funderburk and Syphax, 1969; Quimet-Oliva and Hebert, 1974; Threatt and Appelman, 1973). Sartorius *et al.* (1977) have described elegant improvements in the technique using fine, flexible cannulae.

The examination is carried out with the patient supine and it is important to reassure her that the procedure will cause the minimum of trauma and discomfort. A good light is essential. The nipple should be cleaned with a suitable aqueous antiseptic solution and minimal palpation used to identify the affected duct. Examination seems easier when the duct is not empty of its discharge. A fine, oo lachrymal probe lubricated with anaesthetic gel (2% lignocaine) is used to dilate the duct orifice gently.

Fig. 7.3 (a) Normal ductogram. (b) The ductal filling defect has the appearance of a single intraduct papilloma but histological examination showed a well-differentiated intraduct papillary carcinoma.

This will permit the subsequent introduction of a fine nylon catheter which should have been previously filled with contrast medium (Conray 280 diluted to 50% with normal saline). The system should contain no air bubbles. Injection of contrast should be carried out slowly and should not cause discomfort; the total volume injected will be in the order of 0.5–1.0 ml. A sensation of fullness may be noted in the breast but pain is a symptom of extravasation and the injection should be stopped.

At the completion of injection a seal of collodion or similar material ('Nobecutane') is applied to the duct orifice before and during removal of the catheter. Mammography is then carried out in the standard projections (Fig. 7.3(a) and (b)). Even when extravasation is suspected films should be obtained since they may reveal ductal pathology in addition to confirmation of the leak.

A bloodstained or serous discharge is an indication for exploration of the breast; contrast mammography can facilitate the operative localization and improve the accuracy of pre-operative diagnosis. A negative or unsuccessful ductogram does not alter the need for biopsy.

BIOPSY OF IMPALPABLE BREAST LESIONS

The definitive diagnosis of an abnormality in the breast is made by the pathologist and is based on the naked eye and microscopic anatomy of the biopsy obtained by the surgeon. The incision for the biopsy will depend on the site of the lesion within the breast and on the site of any localizing percutaneous needle left *in situ* by the radiologist.

The patient will be supine on the operating table and the operation will generally be carried out under general anaesthesia. If the co-ordinates are being planned by the surgeon with plain films and without localizing needles, it is important to remember the distortion which occurs during cranio-caudad and medio-lateral compression. The surgeon should measure the distance above the nipple centre on the lateral projection (Fig. 7.4) and draw this (M) on the patient's laterally compressed breast. He should then measure the distance lateral to the nipple centre on the cranio-caudad projection (N) and transfer this to the patient's breast compressed in the cranio-caudad manner. This method of triangulation should locate and identify the position for an incision which should usually be circumferential. Radial incisions in the upper half of the breast may not heal in a very aesthetic way, but at the level of the nipple or below, a radial incision may be more appropriate.

Careful haemostasis should be achieved with the minimum of diathermy, a diathermized vessel in the breast produces a palpable lesion which can be confusing. The breast tissue should be divided in the line of the incision down to the pectoral fascia; this permits careful palpation of breast tissue between thumb and finger above and below the division. Many radiological abnormalities which have been impalpable up to this point are related to a subtle change in consistency which can now be felt.

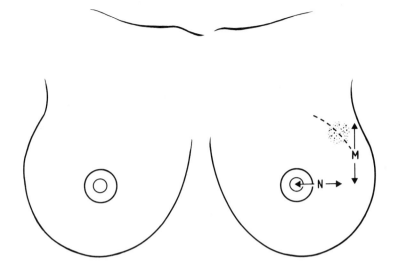

Fig. 7.4   Surgical localization of
impalpable mammographic
abnormality. M=distance of lesion
above nipple transferred from
mammogram to the breast during
lateral compression. N=distance of
lesion lateral to nipple during supero-
inferior compression.

The biopsy specimen selected is marked with a radio-opaque suture and
sent for specimen radiology. The mammograms and the specimen
radiograph should be seen by the radiologist to confirm that the
radiologically abnormal area has been removed. If the abnormality is not
present further biopsies will be necessary, but if the abnormality has been
completely excised the surgeon may obtain haemostasis and close the
wound. Again it is important to stress that excessive use of the diathermy
should be avoided until the specimen radiograph is positive.

Many radiological lesions, especially those containing calcification
without an associated mass, do not lend themselves to frozen section and,
as a general rule, better histological assessment will result from multiple
paraffin sections taken by a pathologist comparing the specimen with the
radiograph.

Excision of a single discharging duct is facilitated by spraying the nipple
with a plastic adhesive dressing such as Nobecutaine pre-operatively. This
seals the duct and ensures that it will be dilated and detectable at
operation. This is carried out under general anaesthetic with the patient
supine. The duct is cannulated with a lachrymal probe. A circumareolar
incision is made in the appropriate quadrant and the centre of this incision
is carried radially towards to probe. With careful haemostasis and
retraction of each triangular areolar flap the major duct is isolated and
ligatured with fine silk. The duct is then dissected into the breast so that
the segment drained by that duct is excised in continuity with the duct.
This specimen should be allowed to fix in Formal saline before dissection
by the pathologist. Papillary intraductal lesions are best examined after
fixation so that their cellular activity and the relation of their base to the
duct wall is properly assessed.

The wound should be closed so that the defect is obliterated by the judicious use of absorbable suture and drainage which should probably be of a suction type. The skin and areolar incisions should be apposed with fine interrupted monofilament nylon or prolene assisted by adherent ('Steristrip') strip dressings. Suction drains after breast biopsies can usually be removed within 12–24 hours and may not be necessary for small superficial biopsies.

8 CYTOLOGICAL INVESTIGATION

P.A. Trott

INTRODUCTION

The role of cytopathology in the diagnosis of breast disease is concerned with the examination of cells seen in nipple discharges and those aspirated from solid and cystic lesions using a fine needle. The former is a well established diagnostic test for carcinoma of the larger ducts, with or without Paget's disease of the nipple, presenting with a bloodstained discharge, but aspiration cytology is a newer technique which is now finding its place in the breast surgeon's diagnostic armamentarium.

In recent years the place of the rapid 'frozen' section in the diagnosis of breast cancer has become diminished in importance and has been replaced by increasing emphasis on pre-operative diagnosis using a combination of clinical examination, mammography and either biopsy, using a wide bore cutting needle or aspiration cytology using a narrow hypodermic needle with a dividing edge, rather than attempt to combine tissue diagnosis and mastectomy at one operation. This change of emphasis is the result of three main factors, firstly the realization that perhaps less radical surgery will give equal or even improved survival as well as less postoperative morbidity, secondly the development of more reliable tests for metastatic disease thereby making extensive surgery unnecessary, and finally the increasing tendency to involve the patient herself in the decision about the best method of treatment thus making accurate pre-operative diagnosis very important.

NIPPLE DISCHARGE SMEARS

The microscopic examination of nipple discharge smears shows a variety of cells including those from duct epithelium, inflammatory cells and red blood cells. The best technique for collecting the fluid is to gently squeeze the nipple, noting the position on the nipple of the discharging duct, and then to place one end of a microscope slide on the nipple and make a thin film by smearing the discharge along the slide. The number of cells obtained is usually small and they dry quickly to enable good quality staining by the Romanowsky technique (similar to that used in a blood film). In a case of Paget's disease of the nipple the excoriating lesion may be quite dry and moistening the surface with a saline swab will encourage cells to exfoliate.

It is important to record the colour of nipple discharge fluid because papillomas, intraduct carcinoma and the rarer intraduct papillary carcinomas usually produce a blood-stained discharge. The commoner clear or serous discharge originates in a subareolar cyst and the cells appear similar to those seen in needle aspirates from cysts elsewhere in the breast. They consist of large 'foam' cells which are former cuboidal epithelial cells shed into the cyst lumen and swollen by the hypertonic fluid, as well as a few apocrine cells and clusters of cuboidal epithelial cells. Occasionally the foam cells have become facultative histiocytes and contain haemosiderin pigment indicating former haemorrhage.

When several clusters of large duct cells are seen in a nipple discharge smear the presence of a papilloma or papillary carcinoma should be considered. The definitive distinction between these two neoplasms is a histopathological one and when either of these tumours is suspected the patient should have an exploration of the appropriate duct and excision biopsy. From an analysis by Dr F. Nardi (not published) of nipple smears from 203 patients examined in the cytopathology department of this hospital, 81 cases had a biopsy or other surgical procedure providing material for histopathological examination (see Table 8.1). Twelve

Table 8.1   Histopathological diagnoses of 81 cases having nipple smears examined.

Histopathology		Cytopathology		
		Carcinoma	Papilloma	BMD
Carcinoma	12	6	0	6
Papilloma	32	2	12	19
Benign Mammary Dysplasia	37	1	1	35
Totals:	81	9	13	60

carcinomas were identified, half of which had carcinoma cells in their nipple discharges. Three other patients exfoliated cells resembling carcinoma, two of these did indeed have a papillary intraduct lesion identified as an intraduct papilloma histologically, but the other was from a woman with a clear discharge and florid benign mammary disease in which duct ectasia was a component and in whom the reactive appearances of the cells were misinterpreted. The sensitivity and specificity of the examination of nipple discharge smears for carcinoma cells is not high but when combined with clinical examination and observation of the consistency and colour of the discharge together with mammography it has a place in the diagnosis of subareolar breast disease. The study also revealed that 8 of the 12 carcinoma cases had bloodstained discharges but 55 other women with bloody discharges had benign disease.

The smears from Paget's disease of the nipple will show a variety of large irregular pleomorphic cells (Fig. 8.1) with hyperchromatic nuclei which can confirm the clinical diagnosis of that lesion.

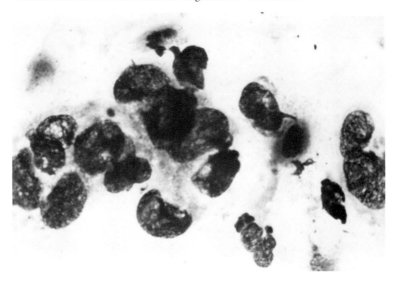

Fig. 8.1 Nipple smear from a case of Paget's disease of the nipple. Giemsa × 1300.

ASPIRATION TECHNIQUES

A good technique in needle aspiration cytology is as important as a good radiographic technique in diagnostic radiology. Without the cells stained properly on a slide no interpretation of their appearance can be made. Of course some breast lesions have a fibrous consistency and few cells will be aspirated but cancers generally are cellular and the inability to aspirate much material by someone with a good technique suggests a benign lesion. In Scandinavia and other European countries the patient is referred to the cytology clinic where a cytopathologist examines the lump and aspirates it as well as looking at the slides later in the day. This is the most efficient way of using the technique and this approach is reflected in the good results from these institutions. No counterpart to the department of clinical cytology exists in this country or the USA although more often pathologists themselves are asked to see patients in out-patients or the wards to aspirate a palpable tumour. In this hospital the vast majority of breast needle aspirates are done by clinicians and there are two advantages to this. Firstly more patients can be aspirated than by having them referred to a pathologist and secondly more information about the nature of the tumour can be discovered by the clinicians from the feel of the needle as it passes into the tumour. The gritty consistency of a carcinoma equivalent to the classical 'unripe-pear'-like feel, familiar to the surgical pathologist who examines the specimen, can be appreciated and provides an additional clinical sign for discerning clinicians. On occasions a lesion thought to be solid on xeroradiography will turn out to be cystic when needled.

The technique favoured in this hospital requires a 10 ml syringe and a 21- or 23-gauge hypodermic needle. The tumour is gripped between the index finger and thumb of the left hand (in a right-handed person) and the tip of the needle inserted into the tumour having first drawn a few millilitres of air into the syringe. The tumour is then aspirated using a lot of negative pressure (about 7 ml if possible) and the needle tip moved about within the tumour in order to sample different areas. In most cases of solid lesions no fluid will appear in the syringe and all the aspirate will be found inside the needle barrel. Before taking the needle out of the skin, therefore, it is essential to even out the pressures inside and outside the syringe either by detaching the needle from the syringe or by releasing the syringe plunger. If the plunger is released then the contents of the needle may be expelled onto a slide by the few ml of air initially drawn into the syringe. The needling is repeated 3 or 4 times to try and obtain a satisfactory cellular sample. The cells are smeared evenly on a slide, usually with a second slide, and either allowed to air dry and stained by the Romanowsky technique or are wet fixed and stained with haematoxylin and eosin. In other hospitals a special syringe holder is used in which the ordinary plastic 10 ml syringe can be held and the plunger extracted with a squeezing device. Some operators prefer this instrument but there is much variation in personal preference.

In an attempt to obtain a diagnosis of impalpable lesions found by mammography various devices have been made to needle such an area which may be an opacity or foci of calcification. At this hospital a device for gently clamping the breast was designed around which a measured ruler containing a guide for a needle was arranged so that the relevant area could be needled accurately under radiological control. At the Karolinska hospital in Stockholm the patient lays prone with her breast protruding through a hole in the table and a similar clamp and guide are positioned to allow accurate needling. These procedures have been useful in a few patients for obtaining cells for cytodiagnosis.

Cytological appearances of cells aspirated from benign and malignant lesions

The number of cells aspirated from a breast lesion depends to a large extent on the degree of cohesiveness of the component cells. For this

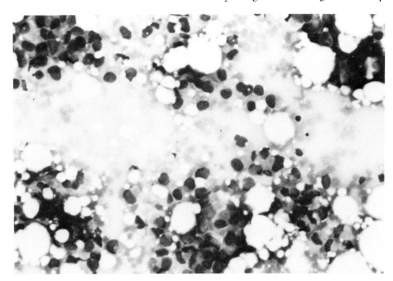

Fig. 8.2 Cluster of carcinoma cells showing a lack of cohesiveness. Giemsa × 329.

reason carcinomas tend to provide more cellular aspirates than benign lesions. The cohesiveness also has important effects on the relationship of the cells to each other on the slide and the presence of tight clusters of cells is a criterion of benignancy whereas in carcinoma the sheets of cells are loose and have uneven poorly-defined borders (Fig. 8.2). Thus it is important to observe the pattern of the smear under the low power objective before examining the cells individually in detail.

In carcinomas generally, the cells are larger, the nuclei are more irregular and there is more pleomorphism than in aspirates from benign lesions. As well as these broad criteria of malignancy there are others that are more specifically applicable. These consist of abnormal chromatin patterns which can be identified whether the staining is by the Romanowsky or haematoxylin techniques and consist of a more granular deeply-stained appearance (reflecting the increased amount of nuclear protein often present) with large nucleoli and often punctate areas of pale staining within the nucleus sometimes called 'intra nuclear oedema' (Figs 8.3 and 8.4). The examination of the nuclear membrane is important because it usually shows a jagged appearance, often slight in degree, but quite different from the smooth outline of the edge of a benign cuboidal epithelial cell. Perhaps one of the most important observations is an assessment of the type and variety of cells present and this overlaps with the histopathological description of a monomorphic appearance of cells in which the variety of cells found in non-malignant conditions has been replaced by an overgrowth of carcinoma tissue. Although in an aspirate individual carcinoma cells will appear pleomorphic when compared one to another the cell type will be similar. One important criterion of malignancy is accordingly a negative one and is emphasized by many cytopathologists. This is the absence of small bare nuclei (sometimes

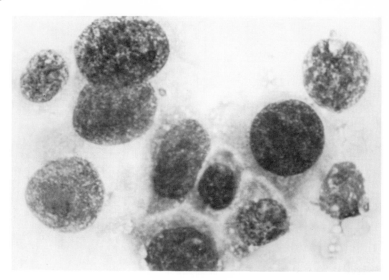

Fig. 8.3 Cluster of carcinoma cells. Compare with Fig. 8.4. Giemsa × 1300.

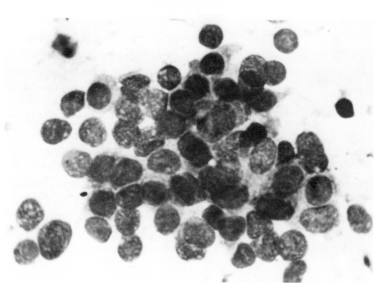

Fig. 8.4 Cluster of benign duct cells. Giemsa × 1300.

called 'sentinel' cells) that often aggregate in pairs and clusters as well as appear singly in benign lesions (Fig. 8.5). They are oval in shape and measure less than 15 μm in maximum diameter and have a single nucleolus. These nuclei are probably myoepithelial nuclei and are numerous in fibroadenomas and other benign lesions but absent in carcinomas. Myoepithelial cells are one component of duct epithelium (the other being the potentially secretory cuboidal cells) and in carcinomas the two types of cells are replaced by proliferating carcinoma cells. In histological sections of fibroadenomas they can be seen within the fibrous stroma where they stain positively for alkaline phosphatase. Their cytoplasm is very fragile

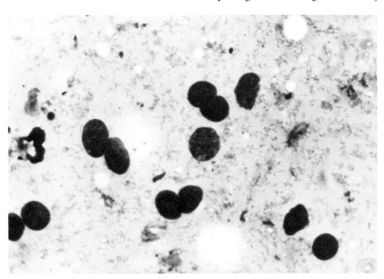

Fig. 8.5   Pairs and single benign duct epithelial cells. Giemsa × 1300.

and often unstained in histological sections. In practical terms when screening a breast aspirate slide, if abnormal cells are identified in a smear in the presence of benign pairs of myoepithelial cells then there must be very good cytological evidence of carcinoma to enable this diagnosis to be made, whereas, in the absence of benign pairs, a lesser degree of cytological abnormality may allow a diagnosis of carcinoma. In other words, because of the limitations of the size of the sample it is unusual (though not unknown) for there to be a mixture of benign and malignant cells.

In the chapter on the histopathology of breast cancer there are some special types described which together comprise about 8% of the total and consist of medullary and mucoid carcinomas. It was emphasized that in their pure form these tumours have a prognosis better than conventional ductal carcinomas and these tumours have definite cytological features when aspirated. The medullary carcinoma (so called because of its soft brain like consistency in contrast to hard scirrhous infiltrating cancers with much fibrous stroma) consists of cells with very large nuclei and prominent nucleoli and a background of lymphoid cells in which plasma cells and immature lymphocytes sometimes with mitotic figures can be identified. The aspirate therefore will give a good guide in a large proportion of cases to the histopathological diagnosis.

More certainly identifiable is a mucoid carcinoma in which the Romanowsky stain is particularly useful for demonstrating mucus which stains a bright purple colour (Fig. 8.6). The cells in this type of carcinoma are small and closely packed with nuclei sometimes less than 12 μm in diameter. When these cells are seen lined up along the edges of streaks of metachromatic mucin a definite diagnosis of mucoid carcinoma is possible.

One interesting subgroup of carcinomas has been identified by their

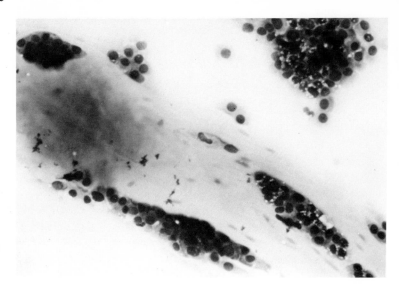

Fig. 8.6   Cells and purple mucin from a mucoid or colloid carcinoma. Giemsa × 329.

appearance at low power microscopy. These tumours have a characteristic pattern when the aspirated cells are smeared on a slide, consisting of diffuse loose sheets of small even-sized cells about 12 μm in diameter. They comprise about 7% of the total breast carcinomas diagnosed in this laboratory and have been called small cell carcinomas. There is some evidence that they originate from the myoepithelium and may correspond to the histopathologist's infiltrating lobular carcinoma. Clinically they are often large tumours in postmenopausal women.

Aspirates from patients with benign mammary disease (known also as mammary dysplasia, fibroadenosis and cystic mastopathy) show a wide range of appearances. The specimens are usually less cellular than those from carcinomas and fibroadenomas and show the different types of cells that constitute these lesions. Thus tight sheets of cuboidal epithelial cells are present as well as myoepithelial cells that are found singly and in pairs within these sheets. In addition other types of epithelial cells are sometimes seen that have undergone metaplasia to apocrine cells, squamous cells, or foamy histiocytic cells such as those seen commonly in cysts. Such a variety of cells will give the clue to the diagnosis.

Foamy histiocytes are also found in fluid removed from breast cysts and are presumably former epithelial cells that have shed into the cyst lumen and become phagocytic. Breast cyst fluid is almost never associated with a carcinoma unless it is bloodstained and the routine cytological examination of clear fluid removed from a breast cyst is a waste of time. Quite often fluid is discoloured and appears blue or green and this is the result of former haemorrhage and haemosiderin pigment can be identified in the cytoplasm of the histiocytes. Carcinomas associated with cysts are of two types; one an infiltrating carcinoma which has proliferated around a pre-existing cyst and shows malignant epithelium lining part of the cyst wall and one that arises within a cyst and has a papillary pattern. These latter tumours have a benign counterpart (intracyst papilloma) in which the papillary clusters of cells aspirated are less irregular and pleomorphic. At this hospital about 1 in a 100 fluids are abnormal and a few of these are carcinomas.

Inflammatory lesions of the breast can be readily identified by cytological examination when the large numbers of polymorphs, lymphocytes and histiocytes are identified. Histiocytes can be very striking and have 40–50 nuclei grouped at one end of the cell. When diagnosing inflammatory lesions care must be taken to hunt for carcinoma cells in cases where the needle has penetrated an area of necrosis within a rapidly growing tumour. This danger also applies to medullary carcinoma in which there is often a large lymphocytic and plasma cell component and the carcinoma cells few in number. The large number of mononuclear inflammatory cells will provide the clue to this diagnosis. In fat necrosis the aspirate is usually poorly cellular but histiocytes and a pleomorphic collection of inflammatory cells will be observed.

Application of the technique and results

That needle aspiration cytology can diagnose carcinoma of the breast is an undisputable fact but the application of the technique as part of the procedure of diagnosis is not widely accepted in this country. Clinicians and histopathologists used only to the examination of paraffin embedded sections remain sceptical that needle aspiration is applicable in out-patients or the surgeon's clinic. However, as stated in the introduction to this section, a pre-operative diagnosis of benignancy or malignancy is nowadays required, which is possible by surgical excision of a lump, needle biopsy or needle aspiration. Excision biopsy provides definitive histopathological diagnosis but requires a local anaesthetic and removal in an operating theatre if palpable and mobile or a general anaesthetic if less surgically accessible. Needle biopsy, usually performed with a Trucut 14-gauge needle, provides a histopathological diagnosis which is less often definitive than the excision biopsy (due to much less tissue being removed), requires local anaesthetic and incision of the skin with a scalpel blade and is often a very traumatic procedure, is uncomfortable for the patient especially for benign disease and often results in considerable haemorrhage. The needle aspiration procedure is a new one in this country and awaits the judgement of published results and accumulated experience.

Table 8.2 shows the results of breast aspirates from 1087 consecutive patients, which were submitted to the cytopathology laboratory from surgical out-patients, arranged according to the cytological result and showing how this is related to the presence or absence of breast cancer. The cases are unselected and include those breast lesions aspirated by experienced and less experienced clinicians such as house officers and

Table 8.2   Accuracy of needle aspiration cytology in 1087 breast aspirates.

Positive	True False	108 1	109
Suspicious	Carcinoma Benign	29 13	42
Negative	True False	664 13	677
No cells	Carcinoma Benign	47 212	259

registrars who have recently joined a firm. This accounts in part for the comparatively large number of unsatisfactory specimens having 'no cells' present although fibrous mastopathy with a small cellular component will obviously yield a scanty aspirate. One aspirate was falsely reported positive and this came from a 41-year-old lady with a fibroadenoma and the appearance of cells was misinterpreted. Fibroadenomas are notorious for mimicking cancer and the few false positive results reported in the literature are usually from these lesions.

Table 8.3 shows the same figures rearranged and indicates the percentage of cancers in which the needle aspirates were positive, suspicious and negative. The 9% false negative result (representing 13 cases from this total of 150 cancers) is similar to the figures in other published reports and may not be as significant as it first appears. Zaijek (1979) found that the cases of breast cancer missed by needle aspiration cytology had a significantly improved 10-year-survival when compared to those that were cytologically positive. The inference being that these tumours are probably smaller and or well differentiated, including some *in situ* carcinomas. The analysis of our cases that were missed confirms this observation although we cannot yet give figures for the number surviving 10 years.

Table 8.3   Accuracy of needle aspiration cytology in 150 breast cancers with cellular aspirates.

Positive	108	72%
Suspicious	29	19%
Negative	13	9%

So what is the place of needle aspiration in the diagnosis of breast cancer? In our hospital it is used primarily in out-patients when the patient first presents with symptoms of breast disease rather than immediately pre-operatively. An analysis of the results of the diagnosis of benign or malignant breast disease using a combination of clinical examination, xeroradiography and needle aspiration cytology in out-patients showed 99% of breast lesions were diagnosed correctly by these procedures in combination and individually needle aspiration cytology was the most accurate. Compared to needle biopsy which can also be performed in out-patients, it has equal diagnostic facility (Shabot et al., 1982). However, the biopsy procedure is not only more uncomfortable for the patient, requiring local anaesthetic and cutting the skin with a scalpel blade, but also more time consuming. At the present time needle aspiration of solid breast tumours is becoming a popular way of diagnosing cancer although some papers report false positive results which are anathema to histopathologists and perhaps should not have been published. Histopathologists also have criticized needle aspiration cytology adversely not appreciating that histopatholo-gical diagnostic criteria do not apply. The technique is considered in this hospital to have a high specificity and rather less sensitivity but with the great advantage of low cost, simplicity, and little trauma.

EAST GLAMORGAN HOSPITAL
CHURCH VILLAGE. near PONTYPRIDD

9 THERMOGRAPHY OF THE FEMALE BREAST

C.H. Jones

INTRODUCTION

Thermography is a method of forming pictorial representations of surface temperature distributions by infra-red scanning or liquid crystal techniques. It is used to investigate breast diseases because breast cancer and some benign conditions alter the surface temperature of the affected breast. Infra-red thermographic scanning systems display within a fraction of a second, surface temperature distributions with high spatial resolution and permit temperatures to be measured and recorded with an accuracy of about 0.2°C. It is a non-invasive, non-contact method of examining patients without any hazard whatsoever. Liquid crystal thermography makes use of esters of cholesterol which exhibit colour temperature sensitivity. When liquid crystal solutions are applied to a blackened surface a given cholesteric crystal will always exhibit the same colour at a specific temperature. A major disadvantage of the technique is that the breast surface has to be blackened – usually with a water base paint. Liquid crystal plates (or plaques) do not suffer from this limitation. These plates can be re-used many times and consist of a thin film support with a black background onto which encapsulated liquid crystals are cemented. The method is easy to use but requires good contact between the plate and the surface being investigated. It is less reliable than infra-red thermography for most clinical problems.

INFRA-RED THERMOGRAPHY

Like all other objects, human skin emits infra-red radiation as an exponential function of its absolute temperature at a rate given by the expression

$$W = \varepsilon \sigma T^4$$

where W is expressed in W m^{-2}s^{-1}, σ is Stefan's constant (5.67×10^{-8}W m^{-2}K^{-4}), ε is the skin's emissivity and T is the temperature of the skin in degrees Kelvin. The exponent of T varies with the spectral range of the radiation being detected. The emissivity is a wavelength-dependent function which describes the extent to which the surface absorbs, and therefore emits radiation like a true black body. A perfect radiator with a surface temperature of about 30°C emits electromagnetic radiation most copiously in the wavelength range 2–40 μm with a peak emission at about 9.5 μm. Although the exact value of emissivity for human skin is not known accurately at all wavelengths, it is generally considered to be approximately unity throughout the spectral region used in IR thermography (Steketee, 1973). A system designed to measure W may be used to measure T or differences in skin temperature (ΔT) providing the infra-red detecting system is uniformly sensitive throughout the appropriate spectral range. In a thermography unit, optical–mechanical scanning devices are used to collect the radiation which is then converted into electrical signals by a transducer, such as a photon detector or a thermistor bolometer. These signals are amplified, processed and used to form an image on a TV tube. The density gradients in the resultant image are a direct function of thermal variations that exist upon the surface when examined. Most medical infra-red scanning systems employ semiconductor type photon detectors such as indium antimonide which responds between 2–5.5 μm, or cadmium mercury telluride (CMT) which is sensitive between 8–12 μm. These detectors are used either in the photoconductive or photovoltaic mode and are cooled by means of liquid nitrogen to reduce thermal noise.

Thermographic equipment

Thermographic cameras may differ in design detail but consist essentially of a scanning system (camera) linked to a display console. The time taken to scan the scene depends upon the camera and varies from a fraction of a second to a couple of minutes. Generally, the slower scanners have better spatial and thermal resolutions, but the faster scanners are more useful for dynamic studies. The accuracy with which local temperature can be measured depends upon machine specification, the surface temperature distribution, and the means by which temperature calibration is achieved. The temperature of an area with a uniform temperature distribution may be measured to within 0.2°C of the true temperature, but larger variations occur over areas in which there are steep temperature gradients. The thermal image can be photographed and this record is called a thermogram. Hot areas can be displayed as white or black (called inverted mode) according to the preference of the user. The black to white level can be set to cover an appropriate temperature differential, usually 10°C for breast thermography so that the temperature distribution over the whole of the breast surface may be recorded. The display console of most imaging systems is equipped with an isotherm function by which a signal is superimposed upon the grey tone picture so that areas with the same

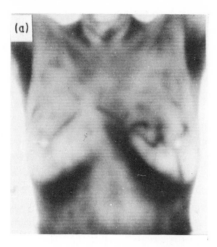
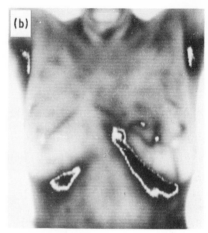

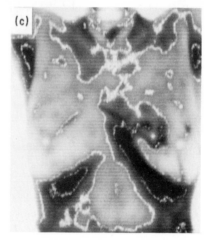

Fig. 9.1   Aga Thermovision thermograms of patient (age 65) with cancer of L breast. (a) Inverted mode; black hot–white cold; white to black 10°C; mid-level temperature 32°C. (b) 34°C isotherm identifying hottest area in L breast. (c) Isotherms indicating 1.9°C temperature difference between breasts.

.emperature are presented as saturated white. The isotherm can be adjusted manually as required within the temperature range of the image. Some systems have two isotherm functions which can be used simultaneously or separately; these are useful for the accurate measurement of temperature differences. Fig. 9.1 shows thermograms of a patient with cancer of the left breast (inverted mode) with a mid-level temperature of 32°C. In Fig. 9.1(b) the hottest area in the left breast is 34°C whereas Fig. 9.1(c) shows the temperature difference between breasts over the areas indicated to be 1.9°C. By judicial selection of the isotherm levels and use of a multifilter photographic camera, or a colour TV monitor it is possible to produce colour thermograms in which each colour covers a certain temperature range. In addition to the use of isotherms and colour imaging, quantitative temperature differences may also be recorded by profile scanning (Fig. 9.2), or by use of an integrator system which averages the temperature over a pre-selected area (Fig. 9.3).

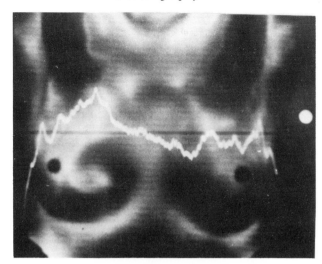

Fig. 9.2   Abnormal thermogram of patient with cancer of R breast (Philips Medical Thermography System). Normal mode: black cold–white hot; black to white 7.5°C, with superimposed temperature profile.

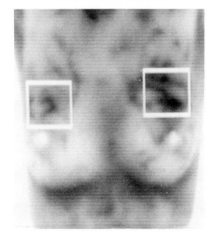

Fig. 9.3   Aga Thermovision thermogram of patient with cancer of L breast with superimposed Aga Integrator 'rectangles' in which minimum, mean and maximum video signals are: R breast 78, 60, 45: L breast 88, 67, 46. (Video level of 50 corresponds to a temperature of 32°C).

Examination of the patient

Breast thermography should be carried out in a draft-free, constant temperature environment. A cool ambient of 19°C ($\pm$ 1°C) is preferable to ensure reliable standardization and operation of the imaging equipment; to cool the skin of the patient uniformly and to reduce physiological variations which might occur with a change in ambient temperature. If the examination room is air-conditioned, the cooler–heater unit must be adequate to balance thermal changes due to heat generated by equipment, personnel and patient as well as any effects due to extreme external temperature changes. The thermostat controlling the cooler should be sited appropriately within the examination area and the room temperature monitored continuously.

Before thermographic examination the patient disrobes to the waist and should sit or lie restfully for about 12–15 min for her surface temperature to equilibrate. Cooling of the patient during this period removes excess heat from the body surface, sharpens up the thermal pattern and helps to stabilize the temperature distribution. It is important that the patient is not overcooled during this period of preparation. She may be examined standing or seated with arms supported laterally or with hands on head, providing she assumes a comfortable position which can be maintained for the examination period. It is, however, important to standardize the procedure so that serial scans for individual patients are obtained under similar conditions (Fig. 9.4).

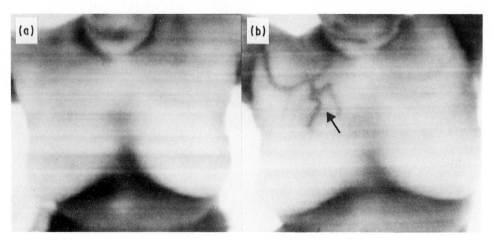

Fig. 9.4   Thermograms of the same patient: (a) patient with arms supported laterally. (b) Patient with arms on head.

THERMAL PATTERNS OF THE HEALTHY FEMALE BREAST

In an ambient temperature of 19°C the surface temperature of the breast is usually between 28 and 36.5°C and covers a range of about 5°C. The temperature distribution over the surface of the breast varies considerably from one person to another, but certain areas are frequently found to have prominent thermal patterns. These areas are: the upper outer aspect of the breast over the lateral thoracic artery which often appears as an area of focal thermal activity, an elongated area radiating medially from the areola overlying the subcutaneous mammary vein which is often between 2–5 mm deep, and an area circumscribing the areola where subcutaneous blood vessels form deep and superficial plexuses. Vessels which course near the surface of the breast carrying blood from deep within the breast result in prominent thermal profiles with widths at half height of 1–3 cm with gradients of between 1–2.5°C cm^{-1} causing an increase in the maximum temperature of the breast of up to about 4°C. Temperature gradients over the first 2 cm within the breast have been found between

$2\text{--}3^{\circ}\text{C cm}^{-1}$, but these and the temperature distribution over the breast surface depend upon the metabolic activity of mammary tissues, the thermal effects of superficial blood vessels, the thermal properties of the epidermis, interconnecting tissue, fat and subdermal tissues as well as external factors such as the environmental temperature.

Changes in deep body temperature such as those associated with diurnal variations ($\pm 0.6^{\circ}\text{C}$) and monthly cyclical variations ($\pm 0.5^{\circ}\text{C}$) can be expected to affect surface temperature values. Furthermore, even when standard cooling procedures are used, surface temperature changes are largely dependent on the physiology of the breasts being examined, vascular breasts cooling more rapidly than those which are avascular. Increases in surface temperature of the breast of about 1°C and intensification of the thermal pattern prior to menstruation have been found to occur in some women; oral contraceptives can cause temperature elevations as well as pregnancy ($1\text{--}2^{\circ}\text{C}$) (Birnbaum, 1966) and lactation (Aarts, 1969). In spite of these temperature changes the overall thermal pattern remains basically unaltered; even after pregnancy the pattern often returns to its original form.

Several authors have classified thermograms of healthy women (Draper and Jones, 1969; Gros et al., 1969; Lapayowker et al., 1971; Amalric et al., 1972). The purpose of such classification systems is to enable identification of abnormal patterns and the estimation of the relative frequency with which thermal abnormalities occur within a particular pattern group. Draper and Jones identified four distinct pattern types and showed that out of a group of 442 healthy women 70% of all thermograms fell into one or other of these groups. Of the women examined 28% had patterns that could not be classified either because of lack of thermal symmetry or because of the absence of any distinctive pattern. Typical thermograms illustrating the four groups are shown in Fig. 9.5: 29% of women had patterns with minimal thermal patterns associated with cold avascular breasts with a breast temperature of about 30°C ($\pm 2^{\circ}\text{C}$): 16% had linear markings and 20% had warm vascular breasts with prominent thermal markings over both breasts with a breast temperature of about 32°C ($\pm 2^{\circ}\text{C}$). About 7% of women had patch-type thermograms consisting of hot and cold areas. The distribution of thermograms in various age groups was analysed and it was found that of women under 30 years of age, 33% were found to have cold breasts whereas 47% of women over 50 years of age had cold breasts; 23% of women under 30 years and 22% of women between 30 and 50 years had warm vascular breasts, whereas only 7% of women over 50 years had warm breasts. The small percentage of women with patch-type thermograms was found to be independent of age. Symmetrical vascularisation of both breasts is rare, so precise symmetry is unusual. Even so, most women who do not have breast nodularity or a localized lump tend to have similar surface thermal patterns over both breasts.

It is evident from Figs 9.5 and 9.6 that many thermal patterns are closely related to the superficial vasculature. There is often a good correspondence between the thermogram and blood vessels that can be

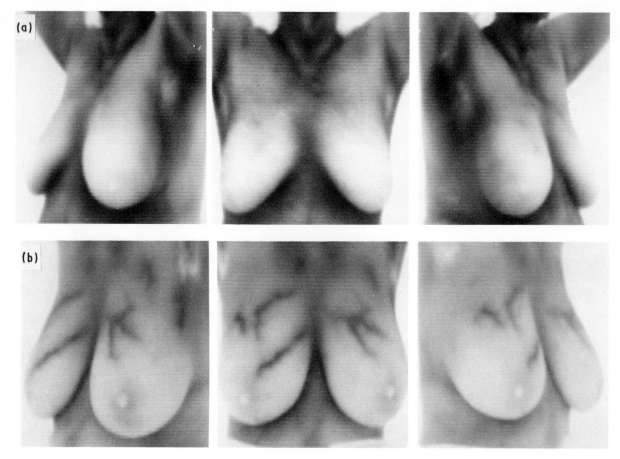

Fig. 9.5 Typical normal thermograms of healthy women (Aga Thermovision, B–W 10°C). (a) Cold avascular breasts. (b) Breasts with linear thermal markings. (c) Warm vascular breasts. (d) Patch pattern type thermograms.

seen visually or recorded by infra-red photography. Each individual has a unique thermal pattern which remains essentially unaltered over a long period of time unless there are pathological changes in the breast or physiological changes influencing breast temperature. Although the precise surface temperature will vary throughout the menstrual cycle the overall pattern remains essentially unaltered even when different types of scanning equipment are used to examine the patient. Fig. 9.6 shows thermograms taken over a 10 year period with three different types of equipment. In spite of the technological developments over this period which have resulted in scanning systems with improved thermal and spatial resolutions, the basic thermal pattern of the patient has remained unaltered. In a group of 205 healthy women examined at the Breast Unit of the Royal Marsden Hospital, London, over a 3–7 year period, 72.6% were

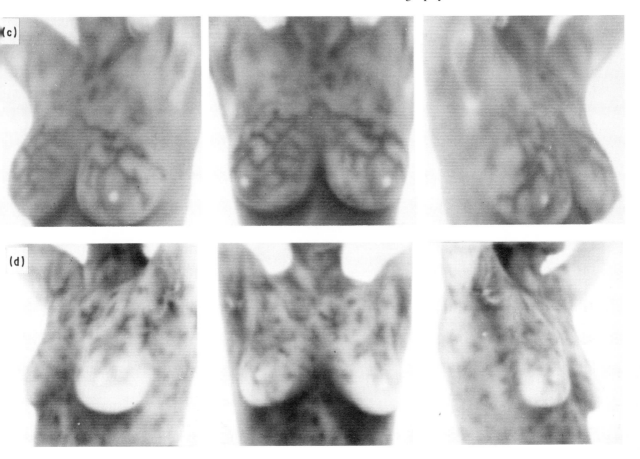

found to have unchanged patterns and a further 18.6% had the same basic pattern but with slight changes in pattern intensity. Almost 9% of the women examined were found to have thermal pattern changes. Most of these changes were identified as being due to menstruation, the use of oral contraceptives, dermatological changes or the development of benign mammary dysplasia.

INFRA-RED PHOTOGRAPHY

Infra-red photography depends upon the fact that radiation in the wavelength range 0.7–0.9 μm penetrates the skin to a depth of about 2 mm. Since blood absorbs this radiation more strongly than the surrounding tissues, when the reflected radiation is focused onto an infra-red sensitive emulsion an image of the superficial vascular pattern is recorded. Massopust and Gardner (1953), and others have attempted to use IR photography for detecting female breast cancer. Jones and Draper (1970) compared IR photography and thermography and found that in a group of

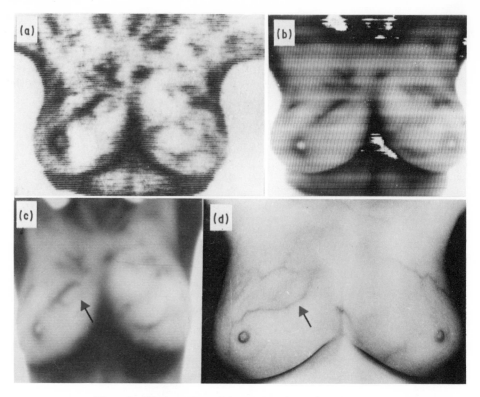

Fig. 9.6 Thermograms of the same patient taken over a 10 year period showing the constancy of the thermal pattern and its relation to superficial vasculature. (a) 1969 Smiths Pyroscan. Thermal resolution 0.4°C. (b) 1973 Rank Thermographic System. Thermal resolution 0.25°C. (c) 1979 Aga Thermovision Thermal resolution 0.15°C. (d) 1969 IR photograph showing prominent superficial blood vessels.

120 healthy women there was good correlation between the IR photograph and the thermogram for 69% of women. In a group of 170 women with various breast diseases confirmed by histology IR photography used alone was less successful than thermography for diagnosing cancer. Out of 60 cases of cancer (30 carcinomas of the right breast and 30 of the left) venous asymmetry was observed in 38 affected breasts and there was usually both an increase in the number of veins and an enlargement of one or more veins. For thermography 73% of right breast carcinomas were suspicious compared with 90% of left breast carcinomas. The results of this investigation suggest that the temperature distribution over the breast is primarily due to vessels carrying relatively warm blood which lie near the surface of the breast. More than half of the malignancies detected thermographically had abnormal IR photographs and this indicates that in these cases the depth of vessels which affect the surface temperature distribution is comparable with the depth of those veins recorded by IR

photography and this can be shown to be between 1.5 mm and 2.5 mm depending upon the skin pigmentation. It was also apparent that in 20–30% of breast cancers the thermal pattern was due to the effect of heat coming from vessels which lie at greater depths. Mathematical calculations show that a 1 mm diameter vein containing blood at 37°C lying at a depth of 10 mm should be readily detectable by its effect upon the surface temperature distribution (Draper and Boag, 1971). In practice the resultant temperature pattern will be complex and will depend upon conduction and convection of heat from these vessels and it is not necessarily the most superficial vessels which cause the most pronounced thermal gradients. For example in Fig. 9.6 the IR photograph shows a prominent vein in the right breast and its associated thermal pattern is insignificant whereas a deeper vein close by has a more pronounced thermal effect.

ABNORMAL THERMAL PATTERNS

A thermogram that shows thermal asymmetry of the breasts is considered to be abnormal if there is:

1. A localized area of increased temperature of at least 1.5°C; this warm area may be focal (hot spot), diffuse, global (that is covering a major portion of the breast) or vascular in appearance.

2. A unilateral increase in heat around the areolar area. The fat layer, a good insulator, is absent at the areola and there is a rich anastomosis of the superficial and deep venous systems in the circle of Haller with the consequence that the surface temperature reflects deep blood flow patterns more readily than other parts of the breast.

3. A generalized increase in temperature of one breast.

4. Thermal asymmetry caused by 'dimpling', nipple retraction or a change in breast contour in the inframammary fold.

Typical abnormal thermograms are shown in Fig. 9.7.

The magnitude of a thermal abnormality depends upon the extent of the disease and the pattern that existed before the disease developed. For example, if the maximum surface temperature of a healthy breast is 36°C then the temperature increase associated with a tumour and its effect on blood flow is unlikely to be more than 1°C since deep body blood is maintained at 37°C. Individually, the abnormal features described above are not necessarily associated specifically with the presence of malignant disease. Benign disease can cause similar thermal changes but in such instances two or more abnormal features rarely occur in concert. The final thermographic assessment is made according to the magnitude, area and location of the temperature asymmetry; attention is also paid to the background temperature distribution over both breasts, the age and hormonal status of the patient. Comparison of thermographic results is complicated by the plethora of criteria that has been used to define

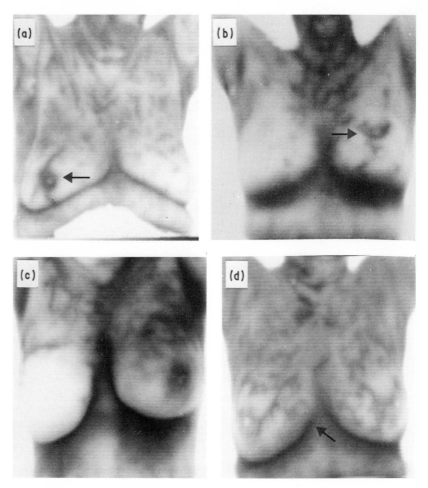

Fig. 9.7 Abnormal thermal patterns of patients with malignant disease. (a) Abnormal thermal pattern around R areola. 3°C temperature asymmetry. Ca R breast. (b) Increased vascularity upper aspect L breast causing temperature asymmetry 1.5°C. Ca L breast. (c) Diffuse, generalized increase in temperature over L breast associated with inflammatory carcinoma. (d) No significant temperature asymmetry but contour change in medial aspect of inframammary fold R breast associated with Ca in lower inner quadrant R breast.

an abnormality and the many different categories of women who have been examined. Table 9.1 illustrates typical findings of a variety of investigators.

Amalric *et al.* (1975) has reported on 4000 women with palpable lumps and found that lipomas, galactomas, and haematomas do not cause a temperature elevation and are frequently associated with a local reduction in temperature. Intraduct papillomas and fat necrosis are sometimes

Table 9.1 Thermographic accuracy in breast cancer diagnosis (a selection from published data).

Source	Population	% Cancers	% True positive (Th + /cancers +)	% False positive (Th + /cancers −)
Hoffman, 1967	1924	1.1	92	7
Dodd et al., 1969	4726	1.2	85	11
Lilienfeld et al., 1969	3518	4.4	72	20
Isard et al., 1972	10055	3.0	71	28
Stark and Way, 1974	4621	0.7	79	13
Almaric et al, 1975	1787	62	74	10
Byrne and Yeres, 1975	2275	6.5	81	32
Jones et al., 1975	1464	25	68	22
	5500	0.7	65	9
Shaber et al., 1976	17500	1.0	70	26
Johansson et al., 1976	1132	13.7	72	47
Raskin and Martinez-Lopez, 1976	1000	5	88	30
Feig et al., 1977	16000	0.9	39	18
	5336	1.0	75	26
Clark et al., 1978	1582	12.8	85	13

associated with a temperature elevation but infrequently. Fibroadenosis, cystic hyperplasia, fibroadenomas and cysts can all cause thermal patterns and temperature changes similar to those associated with malignancy. Inflammatory conditions such as abscesses and infections cause large local temperature increments.

Experience at the Royal Marsden Hospital, London, where 20 000 women have been examined clinically and thermographically suggests the following conclusions:

1. When both breasts are asymptomatic, the occurrence of significant thermal asymmetry is less than 5%.

2. When there is a lump (or localized nodularity) in the breast which is of no clinical or mammographic significance, about 15–20% of these are associated with one or more abnormal thermographic features.

3. 20–30% of benign lumps that are palpable and on the basis of clinical or mammographic examinations require surgery are associated with one or more abnormal thermographic features.

4. About 60–70% of Stage I and II cancers and 80–90% of Stage III and IV cancers have abnormal thermographic features.

5. Non-palpable cancers or cancers less than a few millimetres in diameter sometimes cause unusual, abnormal thermal patterns. The frequency of such occurrences is difficult to assess but this is considered in more detail below.

Details of patients examined at the Royal Marsden Hospital between 1967–72 who had histological verification of their disease are given in Tables 9.2–9.4 (Jones et al., 1975).

Table 9.2 Summary of thermographic and histological results for patients examined and treated between July 1, 1967, and January 4, 1972. Reproduced with permission from the *British Journal of Radiology*.

| | | Number of thermograms | | |
Histology	No. of patients	Abnormal	Equivocal	Normal
Cancer	363 (100%)	248 (68%)	47 (13%)	68 (19%)
Benign	1101 (100%)	240 (22%)	171 (15%)	690 (63%)

Table 9.3 Correlation of thermography report and stage of disease for patients with cancer. Reproduced with permission from the *British Journal of Radiology*.

| | | Number of thermograms | | |
Stage	No. in each stage	Abnormal	Equivocal	Normal
In situ	4 (100%)	3 (75%)	0 (0%)	1 (25%)
I T1 T2 No Mo	152 (100%)	86 (57%)	31 (20%)	35 (23%)
II T1 T2 N1 Mo	65 (100%)	40 (62%)	6 (9%)	19 (29%)
III T3 N1 Mo T3 N2 Mo	108 (100%)	90 (83%)	7 (7%)	11 (10%)
IV M1	13 (100%)	12 (92%)	1 (8%)	0 (0%)
Total	342 (100%)	231 (68%)	45 (13%)	66 (19%)

Table 9.4 Thermography results for 1101 patients with benign histology. Reproduced with permission from the *British Journal of Radiology*.

| | | Number of thermograms | | |
Histology	No. of patients	Abnormal	Equivocal	Normal
Fibroadenosis or cystic hyperplasia	791 (100%)	173 (22%)	129 (16%)	489 (62%)
Fibroadenoma	151 (100%)	21 (14%)	21 (14%)	110 (72%)
Cyst	46 (100%)	6 (13%)	3 (7%)	37 (80%)
Inflammatory conditions	13 (100%)	12 (92%)	0 (0%)	1 (8%)
Other benign conditions	100 (100%)	28 (28%)	18 (18%)	54 (54%)

Factors affecting thermal asymmetry

Although Raskin and Martinez-Lopez (1976) found that an asymmetrical venous pattern is the most common abnormal pattern seen with carcinoma this is also found in benign conditions. Similarly the focal 'hot-spot' produced by some cancers is just as likely to be produced by a benign condition. For example Fig. 9.8 shows thermograms of a patient with an area of focal activity in the outer aspect of the left breast. IR photography shows this to be associated with a superficial blood vessel. Xeroradiography in this case shows no abnormality but demonstrates vascular asymmetry between the upper aspects of both breasts. A diffuse abnormal pattern is more frequently associated with carcinoma than with benign conditions but this is most likely to be associated with large carcinomas.
large carcinomas.

Feig *et al.* (1977) found that thermography was most effective in detecting larger lesions; 83% of cancers measuring 3 cm or more were found on thermography. The proportion of cancers detected by thermography decreased progressively until only 21% of lesions between 0.5 and 1 cm had positive thermograms. However, 54% of cancers 0.5 cm or less were found to have positive thermographic examinations.

Freundlich *et al.* (1968) defined the venous diameter ratio (VDR) as the ratio of the diameter of the largest vein near a lesion compared to a comparably situated vein in the opposite breast as measured on a mammogram and noted that the VDR was significantly greater for cancer than for benign lesions. Feig *et al.* (1977) found that the higher the VDR in a cancerous breast the more likely it is to have a positive thermogram. Furthermore breasts with moderate vascularity as manifested thermographically were most likely to be positive if malignancies were present. Avascular, and very vascular breasts were less likely to produce clearly defined thermal abnormalities. These findings are consistent with the view that for small tumours surface temperature asymmetry of the breast is due principally to differences in blood flow patterns associated with the development of the tumour. Whether such changes are due to the influence of tumour metabolites or local vasculature or arteriovenous shunting or some other mechanism is not known. Draper and Boag (1971) showed by calculation that the heat generated by a tumour less than 10 mm diameter is insufficient to cause significant temperature elevation unless the tumour is very superficial. For large tumours metabolism might affect the skin surface temperature. This aspect has been investigated by Gautherie and Gros (1976). Conduction and convection of heat depends upon the location of the tumour and the volume doubling time of the tumour: tumours with short volume doubling times exhibit high metabolic heat production per unit volume.

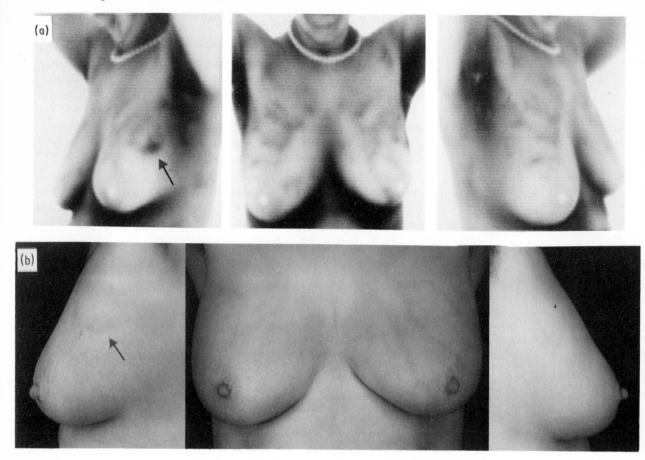

Fig. 9.8   (a) Thermograms, (b) IR photographs and (c) xerograms of patient showing focal area of temperature increase in upper outer aspect L breast associated with normal but asymmetrical vascularity.

The degree to which thermal asymmetry can be relied upon as an indication of the presence of malignancy depends upon the position, size and thermal activity of the tumour, the position and distribution of prominent subcutaneous blood vessels as well as any secondary effects upon these blood vessels as a result of the presence of malignancy. It is difficult to envisage how any but the most superficial tumours may be detected as a direct consequence of the thermal activity of the tumour alone and in many of the thermograms of women with known tumours, the thermal patterns are consistent with increased vascularization of the tumour itself rather than increased cellular metabolism.

It should be noted that the thermogram is useful for comparing the contours of both breasts particularly when serial scans have been taken over a long period. The influence of a tumour in the inframammary fold on

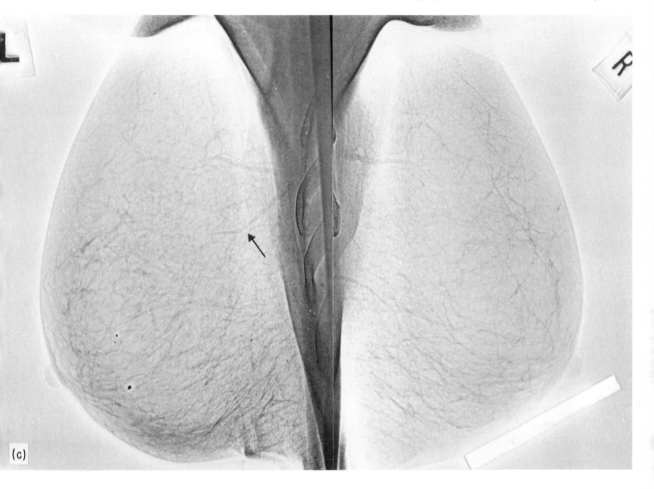

(c)

the thermal pattern has been discussed by Isard (1972) and this so called 'edge effect' is illustrated in Fig. 9.7(d).

It is evident that thermal asymmetry, or a change in temperature distribution is not specifically associated with malignant disease and thermography is of little value in the differential diagnosis of palpable breast disease.

THERMOGRAPHY AND BREAST CANCER SCREENING

Because thermography has both low sensitivity and specificity its value as a screening test has been questioned (Johansson *et al.*, 1976). Revesz (1978) has considered this problem in the following way: it is known that in a population of 100000 asymptomatic women the potentially detectable prevalence of breast cancer will be about 0.5%. If mammography has a specificity and sensitivity of 90% then it will detect 450 of the 500 cancers,

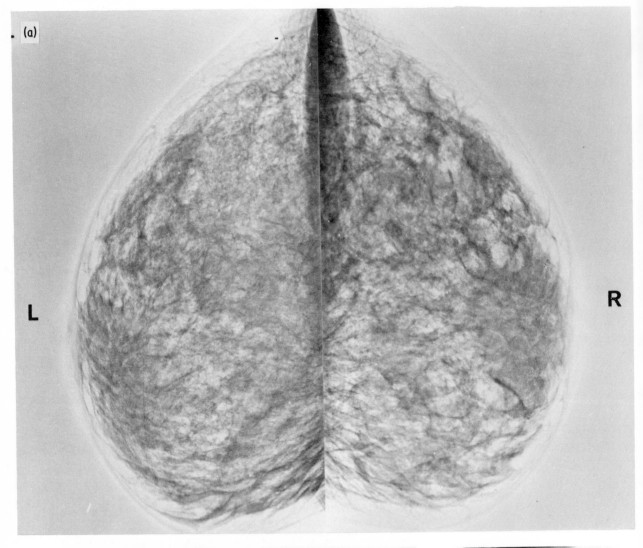

L   R

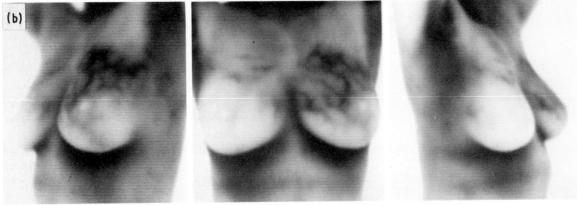

but there will also be an additional 9950 women with abnormal mammographic examinations so that the predictive value (PV) of the test will be 1/23. In the case of thermography under the best possible conditions a sensitivity and specificity of 75% is feasible and for this test the predictive value will be only 1/67. However, when thermography is used as a pre-screening modality so that only the women with abnormal thermograms are radiographed the overall predictive value becomes 1/8.4 which represents almost a threefold improvement over the predictive value of the population with no pre-screening. It also represents a 4 to 1 reduction in the population exposed to radiation and a similar reduction in the costs of mammography. On the other hand the number of cancers missed has increased from 10% to 33%. It must be emphasized that if symptomatic patients were investigated then the prevalence rate would be considerably higher – almost 10% which would result in a predictive value of one half for mammography and initial screening by thermography would then be of less consequence.

The significance of an abnormal thermogram has also been considered by Stark (1976) who found 13.6% of a group of self-selected well women had abnormal thermograms. Out of 744 women, 208 biopsies were performed at the time of the original abnormal thermograms, there also being an abnormal mammogram or clinical findings. Of these biopsies 91% were malignant and a further 44 cancers were histologically proven in breasts with abnormal thermograms during follow up. The time interval from first abnormal thermograms to radiological and, or, clinical indication for biopsy varied from 3–58 months with most cases occurring within 18 months. For these 44 cancers the pick-up rate was 82 per 1000 cases, whereas in a self-selected group as a whole Stark found only 5.8 cancer patients per 1000 and in a high risk group of well women 24.5 per 1000.

Although it should be emphasized that an abnormal thermogram is by no means specific for malignancy, any woman who consistently has an abnormal thermogram should be further investigated. If these additional tests are inconclusive it is necessary to recall the patient for frequent clinical and thermographic examinations. Some of these patients will require careful observation over a long period of time. Gautherie and Gros (1976) found a high rate of cancer in women with abnormal thermograms many of whom were examined over a twelve year period. Fig. 9.9 shows an abnormal thermogram of a patient who has no significant palpable disease and in whom xeroradiography shows benign mammary dysplasia in both breasts but no evidence of malignancy. In the case of localized disease which is either palpable or evident radiographically it is often possible to

Fig. 9.9   (a) Xerograms and (b) thermograms of patient with benign dysplasia of both breasts. Abnormal thermogram L breast.

ascertain whether it is benign or malignant by means of fine needle aspiration cytology. This is less likely to be of value when there is dysplasia in both breasts. Even when thermography is abnormal, it is of small value for locating the precise position of any associated disease so it cannot be used as a guide for aspiration cytology. Consequently patients who have abnormal thermograms but for whom other tests are negative must be watched. Some of these patients might have thermal patterns that will improve by the time of the follow up examination, but those who have persistent thermal asymmetry should be investigated by other methods.

The abnormal thermal pattern of the left breast shown in Fig. 9.9 is associated with asymmetric subcutaneous vascular changes. In an attempt to resolve whether this finding might be associated with malignant disease some workers are investigating the possible use of ultrasound to characterize blood flow associated with breast disease (Minasian and Bamber, 1982). If this work proves to be successful, the complementary use of thermography and ultrasound could provide significant advantages over the independent use of either technique.

LIQUID CRYSTAL THERMOGRAPHY

The application of IR technology to clinical problems has produced high quality thermal imaging systems with very high spatial and thermal resolution. The complexities of such technology are reflected in the high price of commercial equipment. Consequently cheaper alternatives for measuring surface temperature distributions have been sought for many years and it is in this context that liquid crystal thermography has been developed. The use of liquid crystals painted over the surface of a blackened breast has been described by Davison *et al.* (1972). Liquid crystal solutions of esters of cholesterol were selected to respond with a $4°C$ colour temperature range such that the coldest temperatures of the range was red and the warmest temperature blue. The absolute temperature range of response can be varied by altering the solution constituents. Although the technique is uncomplicated it is somewhat 'messy' to apply and unsuitable for examining more than a few women in a short time.

Liquid crystal plate (or plaque) thermography does not suffer from this disadvantage. Apart from cooling and equilibration no pre-examination preparation of the patient is required. The liquid crystals are encapsulated by a special process and then cemented to a pseudo-solid powder (with particle sizes between $10–30 \mu m$) and incorporated in a thin film support with a black background. To obtain a thermal image the plate is pressed firmly against the breast surface. Thermal contact between breast and plate produces a colour change in the encapsulated liquid crystals, red for relatively low temperatures through the visual spectrum to violet for high temperatures. The absolute temperature range of response of each plate depends upon the liquid crystal constituents and several different plates are usually necessary to cover a breast temperature range from $28–36°C$.

Each plate covers a range of about 3°C. A record of the liquid crystal image may be obtained by colour photography.

The method has been used extensively by Tricoire and his associates (1972) and is described in detail by Tonegutti *et al.*, (1980). Interpretation of the thermal image is similar to that of infra-red thermograms and some workers have claimed to obtain comparable results. In spite of its obvious advantages it suffers from two distinct disadvantages: it is a 'contact method' of temperature measurement and pressure between the flexible plate and the breast can influence the very temperature it is being used to measure and, furthermore it is not always possible to obtain uniform contact between the plate and the part of the breast being investigated. The shape of the breast and chest wall greatly influence the area that can be examined.

Local temperature measurements can also be made using strips of liquid crystal film which can be manipulated to contour any curved surface but this method is tedious and more difficult to photograph. Some of these disadvantages have been overcome by means of vacuum contouring with liquid crystal elastomeric transparent Flexi-Therm material (Pochaczevsky and Meyers, 1979).

CONCLUSIONS AND FUTURE PROSPECTS

The value of infra-red and liquid crystal thermography as diagnostic aids is limited by lack of sensitivity and specificity. Benign and malignant breast tumours can produce similar thermal pattern changes; small and large neoplasms can be missed by thermography, a thermal abnormality may have no spatial relationship to the site of origin, and the magnitude of the thermal abnormality is not always related to the size of the neoplasm. However, in the absence of palpable disease thermography can be used to raise 'the index of suspicion' and it is a very useful means of selecting patients for further investigation by mammography. It is completely safe, easy to apply and may be used at frequent intervals in search for thermal changes associated with a developing tumour.

Women who do not have palpable breast disease and do not have significant mammographic abnormalities but who consistently have an abnormal thermogram should be considered to be a high risk group but at the present time there is no justification for taking a biopsy on the basis of thermography alone. In this regard it is with interest that development in ultrasonic breast examinations are awaited. B-type imaging might be suitable for identifying palpable disease but it is unlikely to be helpful for detecting tumours less than a few millimetres in diameter. On the other hand Doppler methods might give additional information about much smaller breast tumours if these affect blood flow patterns in a characteristic way. The application of such a technique in combination with thermography offers hope for improving overall diagnostic accuracy.

The development of thermal imaging techniques in recent years has made it possible to store thermal images and analyse these by computer techniques. These enable appropriate criteria to be determined so that thermal abnormalities can be identified consistently. Comparison of thermal images by computer methods also provides a method of identifying and quantifying changes (Ziskin *et al.*, 1975).

Current technological developments in infra-red scanning include third generation scanning systems with multiple detector arrays capable of fast scanning (50 frames sec^{-1}) and even higher thermal and spatial resolution than are currently available. It is unlikely that thermographic examination of the female breast will benefit substantially from these more expensive systems unless improvements are also made in image stability and processing.

Pyroelectric vidicon cameras are being developed for medical use as cheaper alternatives to traditional infra-red imaging systems. Pyroelectric detectors do not require liquid nitrogen cooling and at the present time are capable of resolving temperatures of about 0.3°C. The basic price of such equipment is about one quarter that of a single element indium antimonide detector system but improvements in stability and quantification of the thermal image will inevitably reduce the cost difference between the respective systems.

Methods of improving the sensitivity of IR thermography as a diagnostic procedure are being investigated and amongst these is the use of microwaves. Body tissue is partially transparent to microwave radiation originating in tissue volumes extending from the skin surface to depths of several centimetres and detection of this radiation with sensitive antennae can be used to measure subcutaneous temperatures. This method has been exploited by Barrett, Myers and Sadowsky (1980) who have used microwave detectors sensitive to 1.3 GHz (23 cm wavelength) and 3.3 GHz (9.1 cm wavelength) radiation to map breast temperature distributions. Although the spatial resolution of such equipment is inferior to that achieved by IR scanning systems the effect of deep temperature variations can be more readily detected. Edrich (1978) has developed a microwave scanning system using 30 MHz and 68 MHz detectors for clinical thermography but at these frequencies only radiation originating in the most superficial layers of the breast is transmitted and the advantages of recording deeper tissue temperatures is lost.

Modification of the surface thermal pattern by heating the breast with radio or microwaves and subsequent analysis of the temperature distribution is also being investigated.

10   ULTRASOUND IN BREAST DIAGNOSIS

T.S. Reeve, J. Jellins,
G. Kossoff and B.H. Barraclough

The most valuable steps taken by the clinician in the diagnosis of breast disease are the clinical history and physical examination. When these two clinical activities have been completed, even by the most experienced clinician, doubt as to the diagnosis may still be present which means that further diagnostic assistance will be needed in some patients. The aids currently available to the clinician for these difficult patients are a second professional opinion, X-ray imaging of the breast by film mammography or xeromammography, aspiration with or without cytology, thermography and more recently ultrasonic imaging. Most patients presenting to their doctor with symptomatic breast problems are concerned about the possibility of breast carcinoma but it is fortunate that most patients with breast disease have some form of benign change rather than malignancy.

In an effort to confirm or disprove the diagnosis of breast malignancy, and this is the crucial factor as far as the patient is concerned, biopsy may be necessary. However refinement of diagnostic aids should lead to a reduction in the biopsy rate with no lack of safety for the patient. Refinement of diagnostic aids may also lead to the diagnosis of impalpable and asymptomatic breast carcinoma.

The development of appropriate ultrasonic diagnostic equipment now allows this modality to play a significant part in the diagnosis of benign and malignant breast disease in those patients selected for this examination following careful history and clinical examination (Reeve *et al.*, 1978). Appropriate use of this technique may allow accurate pre-operative diagnosis or reassurance of the patient without recourse to biopsy.

PRINCIPLES AND EQUIPMENT

Echography shows breast structure and the relationships between the glandular, fat and fibrous components of the breast which enables the clinician to correlate clinical findings and to diagnose different forms of breast disease. Echography does this by the production of multiple images taken at close intervals in either a transverse or sagittal plane. The outlines

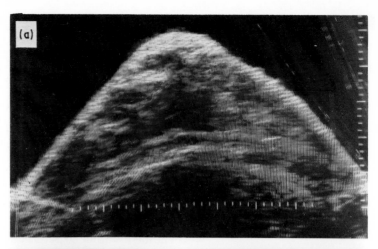

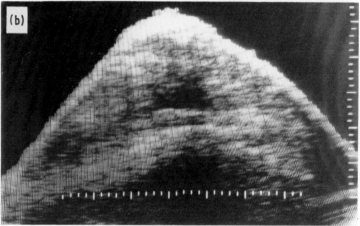

Fig. 10.1   (a) Compound. (b) Simple scan, 39 years. Transverse section. Skin normal in thickness and contour. Virtually no subcutaneous fat. There is dense fibrosis on both compound and simple scans. The central zone of decreased reflectivity is frequently observed in younger and in premenopausal breasts, and probably represents fat. The simple scan is deliberately overwritten to demonstrate this zone better. Note the clarity with which the distinct layers of the chest wall are demonstrated on compound scan.

of lesions are visualized and their internal contents displayed. The total breast content cannot be visualized in the one echogram such as seen in mammography, the tomographic pictures obtained by ultrasound give a better insight into individual areas of the breast and therefore complement mammography. Research scientists of the Ultrasonics Institute of the Australian Department of Health in association with clinicians of the Royal North Shore Hospital of Sydney first developed a scanner using the water bath technique with a single oscillating 4 MHz transducer for this purpose, and from this equipment (Jellins *et al.*, 1975(a); Reeve *et al.*, 1978(a)) was developed the Ultrasonics Institute Octoson (Carpenter *et al.*, 1977) which uses eight such transducers to give high resolution compound grey scale echograms. One of these transducers can be used to form a simple (sector) scan of the breast which may give further information on intrinsic breast tissue detail to that which may be obtained from the compound image.

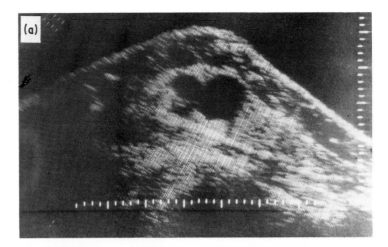

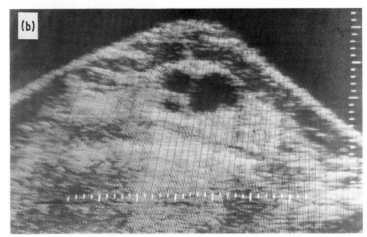

Fig. 10.2   (a) Compound. (b) Simple, 28 years. Transverse section. This echogram demonstrates cystic lesions. The clearly demarcated margins, enhancement deep to the cysts, is more clearly seen deep to the large cyst and is even more clearly seen on simple scan. Refractory diminution in reflectivity is seen at the margins of the large cyst on simple scan.

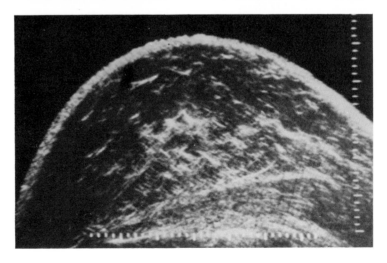

Fig. 10.3   Compound echogram, 35 years. Transverse section. This echogram demonstrates dysplasia in a premenopausal woman. The changes are homogeneous and represent both fibrous and fatty replacement of breast tissue.

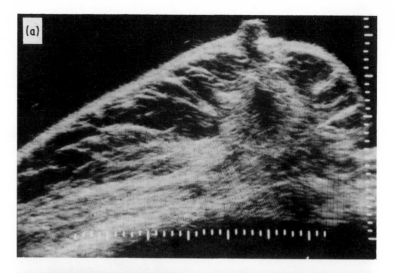

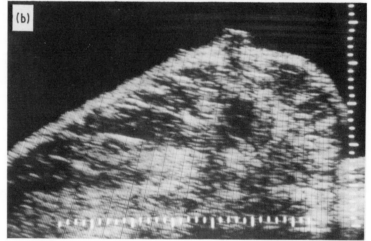

Fig. 10.4   (a) Compound. (b) Linear, 67 years. Saggital section. Skin is normal in thickness and contour. There is a well-defined subcutaneous layer and Cooper's ligaments are prominent. There is a well marked residual breast cone and several residual ducts are noted. On linear scan a shadow is observed to be cast from the nipple. Areas of fatty replacement are scattered through the breast, a central zone of low reflectivity shows some echoes on simple scan and is probably fat. Such findings however warrant mammography and/or biopsy if clinically indicated.

ECHOGRAMS

Despite the non-homogeneity of breast tissue ultrasonic examination can give considerable information not easily obtainable by other means about the composition and intimate relationships of the individual constituent tissues of the breast (namely skin, fat, fibrous and glandular elements).

Tissue pattern recognition allows accurate evaluation of (a) generalized benign changes within the breast, (b) localized solid or cystic lesions, and (c) localized infiltrative lesions.

Echograms obtained using the type of equipment described provide either a basis for immediate decision or a base line record for the patient with 'troublesome breasts'. The quality of the echograms is important and

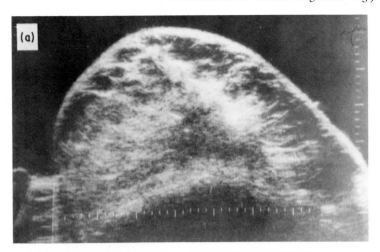

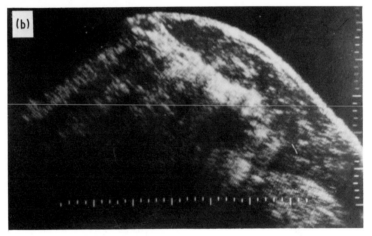

Fig. 10.5 (a) Compound. (b) Simple, 42 years. Transverse section. Skin is normal, subcutaneous layer of Cooper's ligaments are well defined on compound scan. There is a dense breast cone and to the viewer's right there is an area of dense fibrosis. An area of decreased reflectivity is noted deep within the breast which is more marked on simple scan. This was read as being suspicious of carcinoma of the breast and proved to be so. Not all lesions have a classic textbook picture.

This brace of echograms demonstrates the need to have both compound and simple scans of each breast for comparison.

requires significant sonographer expertise (Griffiths, 1978). Figs 10.1–10.6 illustrate significant features associated with both normal and diseased breasts. These are discussed in the following paragraphs.

IMAGE DEFINITION

Normal breasts

The development and changes that occur within the breast throughout life are under hormonal control. This means that the breast has a range of normal appearances depending on the age of the patient and the endocrine stimuli active at the time. The bulk of the breast is composed of glandular tissue which is overlain by a subcutaneous layer of adipose tissue and the whole organ is bounded posteriorly by retromammary fascia and the pectoral muscles. The glandular tissue of the breast occupies a cone-

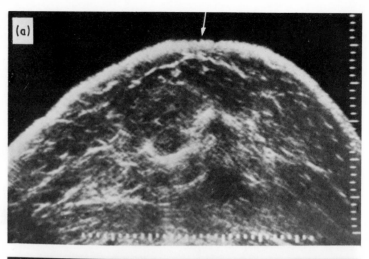

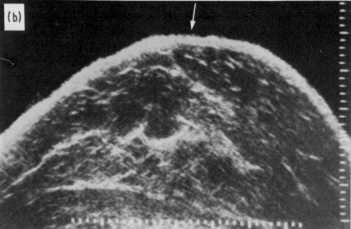

Fig. 10.6   (a) and (b) Compound
echograms, 67 years. Transverse
section. These echograms taken at two
different levels in the breast
demonstrate a distinct flattening of the
skin surface (arrow). This finding
usually implies retraction of skin (not
always seen clinically) when it is
realized that the breast is essentially
buoyant in the water bath. Note the
architectural disruption in this breast
(more marked in (b)), this underlies
the flattened skin and is malignant.

shaped area in the centre of the breast converging on the nipple. In young
adolescent and prelactational patients the central zone of the breast
appears to be more homogeneous than in older groups. This indicates a
normal breast without dysplastic change. The skin is seen as a clear white
line, the layer of subcutaneous fat contains few echoes and is clearly
bounded by the high level echoes of the fibrous capsule of the breast. The
retromammary fascia can be visualized as can the pectoral muscles. The
nipple gives a variable echo pattern and may appear as quite dense tissue or
may be almost echo free.

   As women increase in age and particularly after the menopause the
normal atrophy of glandular tissue leads to its replacement with fat and
variable amounts of fibrosis. Cooper's ligaments become thicker and the
connective tissue components of the breast more dense, so that the normal
appearance in a post menopausal woman may show very little active breast

tissue. In young adults particularly following lactation, ductal activity increases and may be visualized as echo free canals converging towards the nipple.

Tables 10.1 and 10.2 (Kossoff *et al.*, 1976) show the criteria (Table 10.1) for the differentiation of cystic from solid lesions and (Table 10.2) the criteria for classification of normal soft tissues.

Table 10.1   Criteria for the differentiation of cystic from solid lesions.

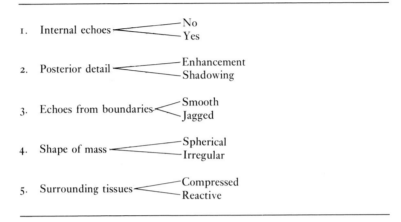

Table 10.2   Criteria for classification of normal soft tissues.

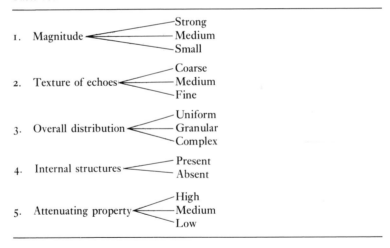

LOCALIZED LESIONS

Liquid-filled lesions

These are readily diagnosed by ultrasound. Cysts and liquid-filled ducts with a diameter of 2 mm or more can be demonstrated with a high degree of accuracy (98%), (Jellins *et al.*, 1977). For the diagnosis of a cyst to be made the lesion should demonstrate complete absence of internal echoes, a perfectly smooth wall, be spherical in shape and situated within breast parenchyma. The other characteristics that verify its nature are enhancement of tissue detail posterior to the cyst which is almost invariable, and refractive shadowing behind the edges of the lesion is useful when present. Particulate matter can sometimes be seen within the cyst depending on the nature of the liquid contained. Following needle aspiration the area where the cyst was situated can be reviewed several weeks later to assess reaccumulation of cyst content but more importantly to review the substance of the breast that had been compressed by the cyst prior to its aspiration.

Fibroadenoma

Such lesions are readily identified in the younger breast. They may be homogenous, but giant fibroadenomas usually show a lobulated internal structure which may be disorganized. The magnitude of echoes of these lesions are usually small to medium, texture of the echoes is fine, the overall distribution tends to be uniform and the attenuating properties of the lesion are low. A feature of fibroadenomata is that the anterior wall of the lesion is often defined by a strong band of high level echoes. In older and more dysplastic breasts which contain more fat the identification of fibroadenomata may be more difficult.

Diffuse benign conditions

In patients with this type of pathology the factors to be noted on each echogram are the degree and extent of active remaining breast tissue, the presence of ductal activity, the degree of fibrosis or fatty infiltration of breast tissue and the general texture and pattern of disorganization of the stromal tissues of the breast. It is mandatory for optimal tissue pattern recognition to compare the breast of the opposite side.

Benign mammary dysplasia

The changes noted in this condition by the clinician may vary from a thickened area in the breast to frank lumpiness and this condition is often associated with mastalgia. It is often difficult to identify specific types of dysplastic change within a breast however echography is a tomographic technique with multiple echograms being taken at close interval, (2–5 mm) in both sagittal and transverse planes. This allows the pattern of the breast architecture to be recognized and its component parts identified. Echograms of younger women with dense breasts reveal quite marked glandular tissue which contrasts clearly with the layer of fat lying beneath the skin. Ducts may be prominent and are seen to converge towards the nipple. The exact significance of excessive ductal presence is unclear, however it does appear that this is seen in the more aggressive types of dysplasia and this may alert the clinician to the possibility of premalignant change. The older patient with benign mammary dysplasia may show variable amounts of breast parenchymal activity associated with fibrosis and fatty infiltration (Jellins *et al.*, 1975(a) and (b); Kobayashi, 1978).

Infiltrating lesions

The presence of breast carcinomata as small as 1 cm in diameter can be recognized and diagnosed with an accuracy of 90% (Jellins *et al.*, 1975(a)). Infiltrating duct carcinoma is the most clearly delineated malignancy, however all types of breast carcinomata greater than 1 cm in diameter can be recognized as specific lesions. Usually their margins are poorly defined with an uneven 'jagged' appearance due to infiltration into surrounding tissue. The contents give rise to low level echoes and up to 60% of carcinomas cause significant attenuation of sound producing posterior shadowing which is usually more easily seen on simple scan. The posterior shadowing may be more readily identified by simple scans taken at different angles (Jellins *et al.*, 1975(a)). If a tumour appears to have a diameter of 1 cm on a single echogram one would expect this same lesion to be visualized on at least four other echograms if they are taken at 2 mm intervals. The most important single criteria in the recognition of breast malignancy is the disorganization which the lesion causes within the fibrous tissue pattern of the breast stroma. Shortening of Cooper's ligaments may give rise to skin dimpling and in more advanced lesions the skin may be thickened or protrude in the region of the lesion. The nipple may be inverted. If the lesion is situated in the deeper layers of the breast the retromammary fascia instead of being shown as a distinct linear region of high level echoes may be interrupted by the infiltration of the tumour. Lesions smaller than 1 cm in diameter have been recognized but confidence in the diagnosis of smaller lesions must be less as the resolution of the equipment allows the visualization of clearly defined lesions to a limit of 2 mm for liquid (Jellins *et al.*, 1977) and 5 mm for solid lesions (Reeve *et al.*, 1978b) and ill-defined lesions such as malignant tumours must approach 1 cm in size before recognition can be achieved with any degree of confidence. If an infiltrating lesion is larger than 2 cm in diameter it tends to lose its localized nature and more generally disorganizes breast architecture. The characteristics shown by smaller lesions are not always present. The echo content is usually of low level but the intensity of the echoes may be less uniform, the boundaries are less well-defined and the jagged appearance of the boundaries may not be present. In these larger lesions attenuation of posterior detail is usually absent and the lesion may traverse the whole breast from retromammary fascia to overlying skin or nipple (Kossoff *et al.*, 1978). The more cellular medullary carcinoma of the breast does not follow the usual pattern of breast carcinoma and tends to have a more

Table 10.3 Summary of ultrasonic findings on breast echograms.

Lesion	Internal echoes	Posterior detail	Boundary echo	Shape of mass	Attenuation	Minimal size detectable	Adjacent structures
Fibroadenoma	Homogeneous small medium magnitude fine texture	Usually no change, may occasionally enhance	Smooth	Spherical	Normal	10 mm	Compression heavy boundary echo
Cysts	Absent	Enhanced	Smooth	Spherical	Nil	2 mm	Compression
Diffuse benign	Irregular strong magnitude coarse texture	Unaffected	Irregular	Irregular	Normal		Normal
Intraduct carcinoma	Low level coarse texture	Shadowing common	Jagged	Irregular	High attenuation	10 mm	Skin dimpling and thickening Cooper's ligament nipple inversion
Medullary carcinoma	Low level fine	Enhanced on occasions	Irregular	Irregular	Variable	10 mm	Skin dimpling and thickening Cooper's ligament nipple inversion
Fat necrosis	Low level	Shadow occasionally	Slightly irregular	Variable	Medium	10 mm	Nil

uniform internal content and greater definition of boundaries.

The interplay between history and physical examination and imaging techniques has been well demonstrated at the Sydney Square Diagnostic Breast Clinic (Croll, 1980), where 30 breast cancers were demonstrated in 1000 women who presented for breast assessment. One patient with frank chest wall recurrence of breast carcinoma was omitted from further calculations. Of the remaining 29 patients 27 had breast echograms as well as mammography and clinical evaluation. There were 4 of these 27 patients in whom the ultrasound study made a significant contribution, in 2 of these the mammograms were non specific. However, all 4 patients had 2 positive results from the 3 modalities used to study the breast. Ultrasound allowed a correct diagnosis in 22 of 27 patients (81%) and 2 patients had positive mammography and ultrasound in impalpable lesions, suggesting that sensitivity of the method is increasing.

This study exemplifies the desirability of having both ultrasound and mammography available in any given centre. They together can help reinforce the history and physical examination. It should be noted furthermore that ultrasonic studies may be repeated without risk whenever needed in the follow up situation (Table 10.3). It is of course

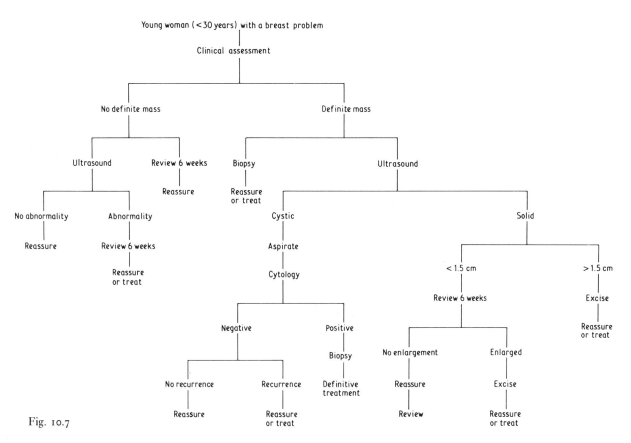

Fig. 10.7

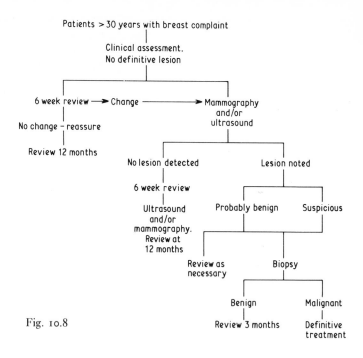

Fig. 10.8

conceded that on occasions the patient's history and the clarity of the problem in physical examination may predicate biopsy without further ado, it may also be useful to review the patient at a different stage of the menstrual cycle before reaching a final decision.

The overruling factor must be the clinical decision, the images are guides and with careful assessment should lead to the clinician being able more frequently to reassure patients. The biopsy remains the important arbiter when any doubt persists.

CONCLUSIONS

The role of ultrasound in the diagnosis of breast disease is gradually being defined (Jellins *et al.*, 1982). Cystic lesions of 2 mm in diameter can be accurately diagnosed as can the presence of a carcinoma 1 cm in diameter and these diagnoses can be made with a high level of confidence. The value of ultrasound in the assessment of patients with diffuse benign disease is being increasingly recognized because the pattern of nodular breast tissue and its intimate structure can be accurately identified and can be reviewed frequently without any danger to the patient. This may be particularly important in younger women and in women with dense breast tissue where imaging can be requested without any anxiety relating to ionizing irradiation. The information obtained using this modality of investigation supplements the information gained by history and clinical examination and is both different and complementary to that obtained by other imaging

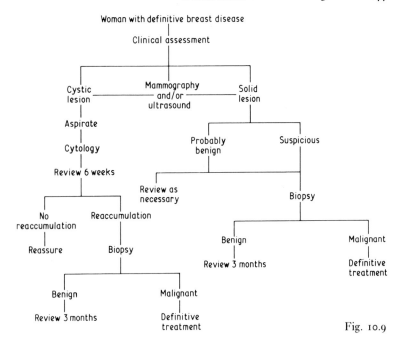

Fig. 10.9

Table 10.4   A suggested plan for following patients at high risk for breast cancer or patients with dense nodular breasts.

1. Clinical assessment
2. Ultrasound and mammography (baseline)
3. Clinical review 6/12 + ultrasound if indicated
4. Clinical review – ultrasound and mammography at 12 months, and then sequence at appropriate times

techniques. The place where ultrasound can be useful in the management of patients with breast disease is indicated in Figs 10.7–10.9 and Table 10.4, they are constructed on the understanding that high quality ultrasound is available.

ACKNOWLEDGEMENT

The authors acknowledge their indebtedness to Dr Joan Croll of the Sydney Square Diagnostic Breast Clinic for Figs 10.3 and 10.6 and for her cooperation in giving details of screening data. The authors also acknowledge the continuing support in their work on ultrasonic study of the breast from the Romaciotti Foundation.

11

DIAGNOSIS IN CLINICAL PRACTICE

J.A. McKinna and J. Davey

The diagnosis of breast disease is dominated by two questions:

1. Does the patient have breast cancer? And if not,

2. Does she have a benign condition for which there is an effective treatment?

The techniques used to answer these questions have been described in the foregoing chapters, they apply to two quite different groups of women, those with symptoms of breast disease and those who are apparently well but attend for screening to rule out breast cancer. The approach to investigation is different for each group. In both circumstances, investigation is best carried out in a particular order. The history and clinical examination are mandatory with additional information from selected special investigations. Which investigations to use depends upon the resources and expertise available so that it is possible to have a number of schemes, equally good in making an accurate diagnosis, but involving quite different techniques. Fig. 11.1 shows a scheme suitable for women with breast symptoms or signs using a sequence of clinical examination supplemented by mammography, fine needle aspiration and biopsy. It has been drawn in such a way as to illustrate a logical order in the examination of women who complain of a lump, pain in the breast or nipple discharge. Other, less common, symptoms such as changes in the nipple, a dimple in the skin, a change in the shape of the breast or a lump in the axilla are of such serious portent that all patients with these symptoms require full investigation, the objective being the diagnosis or exclusion of carcinoma.

The accurate diagnosis of benign breast disease is important in those conditions producing symptoms for which there is an effective treatment. Whilst it will be sufficient for many women simply to be reassured that they do not have any evidence of breast cancer, there are others who will require treatment of some kind to remove or relieve symptoms; in some cases surgical biopsy may be therapeutic as well as diagnostic.

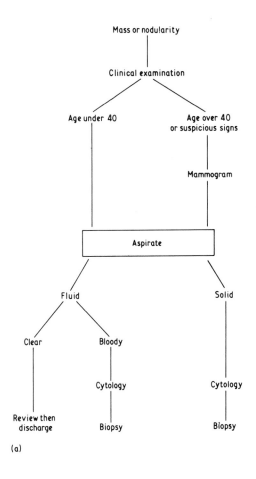

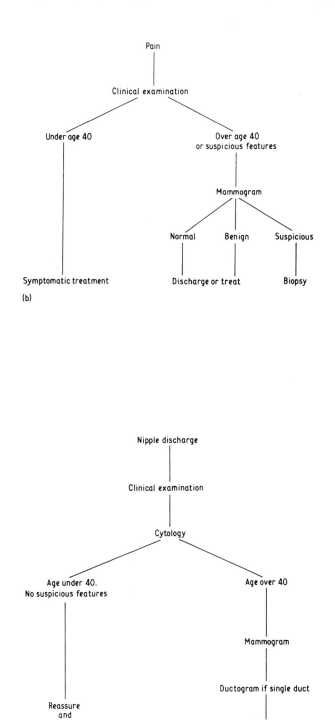

Fig. 11.1 Scheme for the investigation of common clinical situations: (a) a mass, (b) pain and (c) nipple discharge.

EXAMINATION OF SYMPTOMATIC PATIENTS

History

The discovery of a lump in the breast is extremely worrying for any woman and the mental anguish which this causes should not be underestimated. An important point of public education is the inform-ation that the majority of breast lumps are benign.

Localized pain in the breast is usually a symptom of benign disease, but, it is also seen as a presenting feature in 20% of carcinomas. Cyclical mastalgia, which is commonly bilateral but which may affect one breast more than the other, is such a frequent event that it might be regarded as a physiological phenomenon. When it is associated with firm nodularity of the breast biopsy usually demonstrates fibroadenosis or some other aspect of benign mammary dysplasia.

Discharge from the nipple may be blood-stained or serous and of various colours including white, brown and green. A coloured discharge usually comes from cystic disease communicating with the major duct system and pressure on the nipple will indicate that the discharge comes from several duct orifices. Blood-stained discharge, or a serous discharge which is positive to chemical testing for blood, usually originates from papillary intraduct pathology. Single papillary duct lesions are usually benign, multiple lesions may be benign but premalignant, or, frankly malignant.

Other symptoms such as nipple retraction, eczema or Paget's disease of the nipple, change in the shape of the breast, dimpling of the skin with or without a lump in the axilla are more likely to be due to breast cancer and will require further investigation.

Rarely, a patient may present with metastatic breast carcinoma and an asymptomatic, undetected primary tumour in the breast. Conversely, of course, it is important to examine the woman with known breast cancer for possible metastases and it is important to ask about such symptoms as bone pain, sciatica and breathlessness.

The routine questioning and examination of women with breast disease is helped by having a check-list of questions which are related to the breast and to her general health. These should be kept as simple as possible so that the examiner may concentrate on the physical signs. Traditionally, this examiner is a doctor but there are many recent reports about the use of trained paramedical personnel in the field of primary breast examination (George *et al.*, 1980; White *et al.*, 1978).

Clinical signs

The mainstay of clinical examination is inspection of the breast in different views and palpation in different positions, these have been described earlier (Chapter 2). It is important to describe the physical signs in a

Fig. 11.2 The TNM staging chart for the breast (*see also overleaf*) of the International Union Against Cancer. Reproduced with the permission of the International Union Against Cancer.

© Copyright International Union Against Cancer 1980.

BREAST
ICD-O T-174

Centre	Case No. Ident. No.
Patient	Reg. Year
Date of Birth	Age Sex Ann. Month

PRE-TREATMENT CLINICAL CLASSIFICATION (TNM)
→ Please check one or more items in each section as applicable. See mimimum requirements for assessment on reverse side

Site and Size of Primary Tumour

Medial ☐   Central ☐   Lateral ☐   Quadrant ☐

Tumour size in greatest dimension   cm

Measured by caliper ☐   By mammography ☐

Supplementary Information

Paget's disease beyond the nipple ☐

Nipple retraction ☐   Skin tethered or dimpled ☐

Regional lymph nodes:
Histologically negative ☐   Histologically positive ☐

Histological diagnosis

Grade

PRIMARY TUMOUR
→ If not assessed, check TX ☐

SIZE	EXTENSION TO SKIN IN BREAST AREA	FIXATION TO PECTORAL FASCIA OR MUSCLE		FIXATION TO CHEST WALL		CATEGORY	STAGE
Pre-invasive carcinoma (in situ) or Paget's disease of nipple with no tumour					☐	Tis	—
No evidence of primary tumour					☐	T0	—
2 cm or less ☐	No significant direct extension ☐	None	☐	None	☐	T1a	I
		Present	☐			T1b	
More than 2 but not more than 5 cm ☐		None	☐			T2a	II
		Present	☐			T2b	
More than 5 cm ☐		None	☐			T3a	IIIa
		Present	☐			T3b	
Tumour Of Any Size				Present	☐	T4a	IIIb
	Infiltration ☐ Peau d'orange ☐ Oedema ☐ Satellite ☐ Ulceration ☐ nodules			None	☐	T4b	
				Present	☐	T4c	

REGIONAL LYMPH NODES
→ If not assessed check NX ☐

HOMOLATERAL AXILLARY NODES		SUPRA & INFRA-CLAVICULAR NODES	OEDEMA OF ARM	CATEGORY	STAGE
Not palpable ☐		Not palpable ☐	None ☐	N0	I
Palpable, but movable ☐	Not considered to contain growth ☐			N1a	I
	Considered to contain growth ☐			N1b	II
Fixed * ☐	Fixed to one another ☐			N2	IIIa
	Fixed to other structures ☐				
* Considered to contain growth		Palpable * ☐	Present ☐	N3	IIIb

DISTANT METASTASES
→ If not assessed, check MX ☐

		CATEGORY	STAGE
No evidence of distant metastases	☐	M0	I
Evidence of distant metastases (specify)	☐	M1	IV

Information obtained: Before admission ☐ At Centre ☐ Examiner   Date   T   N   M   STAGE   G

POST-SURGICAL HISTOPATHOLOGICAL CLASSIFICATION (p.TNM)
→ Please check one or more items in each section as applicable. See mimimum requirements for assessment on reverse side

Site and Size of Primary Tumour

Medial ☐   Central ☐   Lateral ☐   Quadrant ☐

Tumour size in greatest dimension   cm

Surgery: Biopsy: Incisional ☐   Excisional ☐
Partial Mastectomy ☐   Total Mastectomy ☐
Modified Radical ☐   Radical ☐

Gross Specimen:

Histological diagnosis

Grade

Regional Nodes	No.	Size	No. Gross	Pos. Micro
Axillary I				
Axillary II				
Axillary III				
Infraclavicular				
Supraclavicular				
Int. Mammary				

PRIMARY TUMOUR
→ If not assessed, check pTX ☐

SIZE	EXTENSION TO SKIN IN BREAST AREA	FIXATION TO PECTORAL FASCIA OR MUSCLE		FIXATION TO CHEST WALL		CATEGORY	STAGE
Pre-invasive carcinoma (in situ) or Paget's disease of nipple with no tumour					☐	pTis	—
No evidence of primary tumour					☐	pT0	—
≤ 0.5cm ☐ > 0.5 − 1.0 ☐ > 1.0 − 2.0 ☐	No significant direct extension ☐	None	☐	None	☐	pT1a	I
		Present	☐			pT1b	
More than 2 but not more than 5 cm ☐		None	☐			pT2a	II
		Present	☐			pT2b	
More than 5 cm ☐		None	☐			pT3a	IIIa
		Present	☐			pT3b	
Tumour Of Any Size				Present	☐	pT4a	IIIb
	Infiltration ☐ Peau d'orange ☐ Oedema ☐ Satellite ☐ Ulceration ☐ nodules			None	☐	pT4b	
				Present	☐	pT4c	

REGIONAL LYMPH NODES
→ If not assessed, check pNX ☐

HOMOLATERAL AXILLARY NODES		SUPRA & INFRA-CLAVICULAR NODES	OEDEMA OF ARM	CATEGORY	STAGE
Not palpable, no evidence of invasion ☐		No invasion ☐	None ☐	pN0	I
Movable, with invasion ☐	Microscopic evidence (≤.2 cm) ☐			pN1a	I
	Gross evidence (i, ii, iii, iv) * ☐			pN1b	II
Fixed, with invasion ☐	Fixed to one another ☐			pN2	IIIa
	Fixed to other structures ☐				
* See reverse side		Invasion ☐	Present ☐	pN3	IIIb

DISTANT METASTASES
→ If not assessed, check pMX ☐

		CATEGORY	STAGE
No evidence of distant metastases	☐	pM0	I
Evidence of distance metastases (specify)	☐	pM1	IV

Information obtained: Before admission ☐ At Centre ☐ Clinician   Date   AHS pT   pN   pM   STAGE   G

1980 (U.I.C.C. 1978)   **THE INTERNATIONAL UNION AGAINST CANCER**

BREAST

PRE-TREATMENT CLINICAL CLASSIFICATION (TNM)

Minimum Requirements for Assessment; T,N — Clinical examination; M — Clinical examination and radiography.

T - Primary Tumour

Tis Pre-invasive carcinoma (carcinoma in situ), non-infiltrating intraductal carcinoma, or Paget's Disease of the nipple with no demonstrable tumour.

Note: Paget's Disease associated with a demonstrable tumour is classified according to the size of the tumour.

TO No evidence of primary tumour.

Note: Dimpling of the skin, nipple retraction, or any other skin changes except those in T4b may occur in T1, T2 or T3.

T1 Tumour of 2 cm or less in its greatest dimension.
- T1a With no fixation to underlying pectoral fascia and/or muscle.
- T1b With fixation to underlying pectoral fascia and/or muscle.

T2 Tumour more than 2 cm but not more than 5 cm in its greatest dimension.
- T2a With no fixation to underlying pectoral fascia and/or muscle.
- T2b With fixation to underlying pectoral fascia and/or muscle.

T3 Tumour more than 5 cm in its greatest dimension.
- T3a With no fixation to underlying pectoral fascia and/or muscle.
- T3b With fixation to underlying pectoral fascia and/or muscle.

T4 Tumour of any size with direct extension to chest wall or skin.

Note: Chest wall includes ribs, intercostal muscles and serratus anterior muscle but not pectoral muscle.

- T4a With fixation to chest wall.
- T4b With oedema, infiltration or ulceration of skin of breast (including peau d'orange), or satellite skin nodules confined to the same breast.
- T4c Both of above.

Note: Cases of inflammatory carcinoma should be reported as a separate group.

TX Minimum requirements to assess the primary tumour can not be met.

N - Regional Lymph Nodes

The regional lymph nodes are the axillary nodes, the infraclavicular nodes and the supraclavicular nodes.

NO No palpable homolateral axillary nodes.

N1 Movable homolateral axillary nodes.
- N1a Nodes not considered to contain growth.
- N1b Nodes considered to contain growth.

N2 Homolateral axillary nodes fixed to one another **or** to other structures and considered to contain growth.

N3 Homolateral supraclavicular or infraclavicular nodes and considered to contain growth **or** oedema of the arm.

Note: Oedema of the arm may be caused by lympatic obstruction; lymph nodes may not then be palpable.

NX Minimum requirements to assess the regional lymph nodes can not be met.

M - Distant Metastases

MO No evidence of distant metastases.

M1 Evidence of distant metastases (specify, using recommended abbreviations).

MX Minimum requirements to assess the presence of distant metastases can not be met.

POST-SURGICAL HISTOPATHOLOGICAL CLASSIFICATION (p.TNM)

pT - Primary Tumour

The pT categories correspond to the T categories with two exceptions:
pT1a and pT1b are subdivided thus: $\leq$0.5cm, >0.5—1.0cm, >1.0—2cm.

pN - Regional Lymph Nodes

The pN categories correspond to the N categories with the following exceptions:

pN1a Micrometastases $\leq$0.2 cm or less.
pN1b Gross evidence of metastases, subdivided into: i.) Metastases > 0.2cm in 1-3 nodes; ii) metastases >0.2cm in 4 or more nodes; iii) metastases beyond capsule of a node; iv) a positive node $\geq$ 2cm in diameter.

Note: Homolateral internal mammary nodes may be included in the pN3 category, the fact to be stated.

pM - Distant Metastases

The pM categories correspond to the M categories.

Histopathological Grading (G): Record as G1—High degree of differentiation, G2—Medium, G3—Low degree or Undifferentiated, GX—Not assessed.

Additional Descriptors: For recurrent cases, add prefix **r**. For cases having other treatment before surgery, add prefix **y**.

STAGE-GROUPING

Stage	T	N	M	Stage	T	N	M
Stage I	T1a, T1b	NO, N1a	MO	Stage IIIa	T3a, T3b	NO,N1	MO
Stage II	TO	N1b	MO		T1-3a,b	N2	MO
	T1a, T1b	N1b	MO	Stage IIIb	T1-3a,b	N3	MO
	T2a, T2b	NO. N1a	MO		T4a,b,c	Any N	MO
	T2a, T2b	N1b	MO	Stage IV	Any T	Any N	M1

For Statistical Purposes Only					
Date Registered	**Pathological Report**		**Date treatment begun**	**Anniversary Status***	
Primary ☐ Residual ☐ Previous ☐ Recurrent ☐	Primary: Neg, ☐ Nodes: Neg. ☐ Pos. ☐ Pos. ☐ N.S. ☐ N.S. ☐		Initial Treatment Surgery ☐ Radiotherapy ☐ Surg. & Radio. ☐	1 A ☐ D ☐ L ☐ 2 A ☐ D ☐ L ☐ 3 A ☐ D ☐ L ☐	
Date of Death Underlying Cause of Death Associated/Contributory Causes			Other (specify) ☐ None ☐	4 A ☐ D ☐ L ☐ 5 A ☐ D ☐ L ☐ *End of 1, 2, 3, 4, 5, Years	

standard way noting particularly size, site, shape, surface and consistency of masses within the breast, of attachment to the skin or to deeper structures and to record the state of the regional lymphatic drainage.

The clinical features of malignant tumours have been coded in the TNM system. Fig. 11.2 shows the TNM check-list to describe the physical signs found on first examination: care taken at this time is usually well rewarded and on completing the first examination, it is important to make a provisional clinical diagnosis (UICC, 1980). A second clinical examination at a different time in the woman's menstrual cycle when the breast parenchyma is less nodular, may allow a clearer impression of the physical characteristics of a mass.

Special investigations

Which other examinations are necessary or may possibly be helpful to confirm the diagnosis? Although the sequence in which special investigations are carried out may be varied, assessment of the findings should not be taken out of sequence in the final exercise of diagnostic judgement. For example, it is our own practice that women over the age of 40 who have breast symptoms should be examined by mammography prior to the clinical examination. The clinician has the films made available immediately after the first physical examination and may then choose to re-examine the patient if an occult abnormality has been shown on the mammogram. Clinical examination after mammography allows fine needle aspiration of suspicious areas to be carried out without the risk of haematoma causing confusing changes on the mammogram.

The sequence of examinations may vary under different circumstances. A woman of 34 who is not taking contraceptive precautions presents with a one-week history of a lump in the third week of her menstrual cycle. For her, the diagnosis may be made by physical examination followed by fine needle aspiration which demonstrates the presence of a cyst. She should then be re-examined six weeks later at a different time in her menstrual cycle, when mammography would be safe, if the clinician felt that it was an appropriate investigation in the light of residual physical findings, or other indications such as large breasts, or a maternal family history of breast cancer. It is not uncommon for such a mammogram to detect an unsuspected cyst in the opposite breast. A completely different approach would be taken for a woman of 45 presenting in mid-cycle with a one-week history of a lump in the breast which on clinical examination had any suspicious features whatsoever. Here, mammography should be the next investigation. However, the suspicious clinical findings make open biopsy mandatory in such a case even in the face of negative mammography and cytology.

Mammography

Selection of patients for mammography can be guided by working rules agreed between the clinician and radiologist (Andersson *et al.*, 1978 and 1979). It is probably sensible to have a working rule not to radiograph the breasts of women under the age of 40 unless there are specific indications. There has been anxiety about radiation dose and its possibly harmful effect (Bailar, 1976; Simon and Silverstone, 1976). This anxiety may be particularly justified in a screening situation where young women may be exposed to regular breast irradiation at annual or bi-annual intervals without the likelihood of a high yield of serious pathology, but with a considerable accumulated life-time radiation dose to the patient (Hammerstein *et al.*, 1979). On the other hand, efforts to protect a patient from a potential radiation hazard must not diminish the efficiency of the diagnostic procedure (Haus, 1977). An inadequate radiological examination is of no help to the clinician or the patient. Clinical details may help the radiographer to tailor the examination to the patient's problem and will help the radiologist to report on the examination in an informed way. Whilst the lateral and cranio-caudad projections are the usual routine views the detection of mass in an uncommon site may require special views such as a reversed lateral or an extended cranio-caudad. It may be helpful if the clinician indicates the presence of a clinical mass in the breast with a small mark on the skin. The radiographer and radiologist will be able to give their best service when the physical findings are described accurately whilst lack of this information may mar the whole investigation.

False negative results in mammography are related to the density of the breast tissue, the breast parenchymal pattern and the site and size of the primary tumour. A small but easily felt tumour lying within a dense breast may easily be diagnosed by the clinician as suspicious of carcinoma without any radiological features to confirm the diagnosis. The false negative rate for mammography is reduced when the films are read by more than one observer whether these are all radiologists or some are paramedical staff (Golinger *et al.*, 1979).

False positive examinations are less common and are caused by benign conditions, such as sclerosing adenosis and fat necrosis, which may have one or more radiological features more commonly seen in cancer (Egeli, 1979).

When the clinical and radiological information are available, the surgeon must decide if any further test is necessary to confirm the diagnosis. The experienced clinician will do this at the time of re-examination of the breasts with the mammograms. It is not sufficient just to read a radiograph report, it is an essential part of the discipline that the patient and her mammograms should be examined at the same time. An improved standard of practice can be achieved by clinician and radiologist holding regular review meetings to correlate clinical and radiological abnormalities with the cytological and histological results (Bassett *et al.*, 1978; Minagi and Youker, 1968).

Thermography

Thermography does not diagnose breast cancer, or play any part in the differential diagnosis of breast conditions, but it does indicate abnormality in a breast requiring further investigation (Jones *et al.*, 1975). It is a useful and harmless investigation which, if carried out carefully, can give a reproducible pattern for an individual patient. Asymmetry and abnormality of that pattern has been described by Stark (1976) and by Gros *et al.* (1969) as an indication of high risk for the later development of breast carcinoma and a change in the thermal pattern may be an indication of the need for further investigation.

Jones *et al.* (1975) have also shown that an abnormal thermogram has a prognostic value in breast cancer since thermographically occult carcinomas have a better prognosis than those tumours which demonstrate thermal activity. The role of thermography in screening will be discussed later in this chapter.

Ultrasound

Ultrasound examination of the breast, like mammography is not an isolated investigation (Griffiths, 1978). It has a demonstrable role in indicating the difference between solid and cystic lesions (Jellins *et al.*, 1971). The ultrasonic characteristics of a tumour within fibrocystic disease may be more informative than mammography and it is hoped that this investigation which does not carry radiological hazard will add to diagnostic accuracy in the younger woman with dense breasts.

Other investigations

As each new imaging modality becomes available there are workers interested to test its efficiency at breast cancer diagnosis. These include computed tomography, nuclear magnetic resonance, diaphanoscopy and the measurement of the electrical charge transmitted through the breast tissue. At the moment, these are experimental techniques or have not shown any advantage in clinical practice over the more standard procedures already described (Jones, 1982).

Breast biopsy

Ultimately breast diagnosis depends upon the histology of biopsy specimens. Of course, the accuracy of the histological diagnosis is dependent upon biopsy of an appropriate site (Lewis *et al.*, 1976). This is rarely a problem where there is a single dominant mass, but it may be much more of a problem where the mass is part of a diffuse change within the breast, or where the lesion is detected by radiology rather than by clinical examination (Millis *et al.*, 1976b; Nordenstrom and Zajicek, 1977; Becker, 1979; Frank *et al.*, 1976).

Fine needle aspiration of a breast mass detects fluid in simple cysts and it provides further information about areas of solid breast tissue (Kreuzer, 1978; Webb, 1975). The consistency of solid tissue may impart a particular sign to the examining fingers. It is not uncommon for the insertion of a needle into a scirrhous or fibroblastic carcinoma to feel firm and gritty, however, a similar gritty feeling may be elicited by a needle whose point is minimally, but not visually, barbed. Benign fibrous breast tissue may be so dense that it grips and may even bend the needle. Needle aspiration provides an extension of physical examination (Fentiman, 1980).

Fine needle aspiration will often yield tissue fluid that can be made into a smeared preparation suitable for cytodiagnosis (Rimsten *et al.*, 1975; Russ *et al.*, 1978; Thomas *et al.*, 1978; Zajdela, 1979). This may reduce the need for frozen section examination in the treatment of breast cancer. At The Memorial Hospital, New York, where the technique has been used for many years, pre-operative cytodiagnosis of malignancy is made the night before definitive breast surgery. Failure to demonstrate malignant cells indicates to the surgeon that he must carry out a biopsy and frozen section examination before proceeding to mastectomy.

Trott (Chapter 8) has already described our experience of fine needle aspiration, where we use the detection of benign breast epithelial cells to confirm a combined clinical and radiological diagnosis of benign mammary dysplasia. This prevents an unnecessarily high benign biopsy rate. During the time aspiration cytology has been available in our practice, the ratio of benign to malignant biopsies have decreased from 6:1 to 2.5:1.

The ultimate tissue diagnosis is made histologically rather than cytologically (Zajicek, 1979). Satisfactory material for histology can be obtained by wide wall needle biopsy (Tru-cut), by high speed drill biopsy or by open biopsy (Roberts *et al.*, 1975; Elston *et al.*, 1978). The former methods are suitable for the confirmatory diagnosis of carcinomas which are 2 cm or greater in size, but smaller tumours and benign conditions usually need an open excisional biopsy (Shabot *et al.*, 1982).

A high biopsy rate contributes to an overall low frequency of false negative diagnoses, but all palpable lumps do not need to be excised. Cysts containing clear fluid with no residual mass after aspiration are unlikely to be directly associated with breast cancer so that excision is not justified on those grounds. In premenopausal women re-examination after an interval of two or three weeks at a different time in the menstrual cycle is helpful to ensure that the lump persists. In the perimenopausal or postmenopausal patient all palpable single solid discrete masses should be removed, not for frozen section and immediate mastectomy but for histological confirmation of a diagnosis which will already have been suggested by the clinical examination or special investigations. Problems may arise if the palpable lump merges with an area of nodularity, or if there are multiple masses. In these circumstances, even the experienced clinician finds the decision whether or not to biopsy difficult. Occasionally, therefore, the patient requests biopsy to avoid repeated visits for assessment. Where possible, the reason for biopsy should be recorded.

Occasionally suspicious features on a mammogram will be the sole reason for biopsy. Millis *et al.* (1976b) have reported different methods of approaching the biopsy of localized mammographic calcification. Rosen *et al.* (1974) and Rosen *et al.* (1980) have reported series of biopsies for calcification in which the incidence of malignancy was 10–20%. Our own experience of 131 biopsies for impalpable calcification has shown that 33% of the cases yielded malignant biopsies although many were only *in situ* carcinoma (Table 11.1). Occasionally the mammographic abnormality will be increased density or a disturbance of architecture which is apparent on only one view. In these circumstances it may be reasonable to have a follow-up examination after two or three months since the vast majority of tumours which cause these abnormalities are apparent in two planes.

Table 11.1 Specimen radiology and impalpable mammographic abnormalities. A five year experience of biopsies for impalpable mammographic abnormalities.

	Calcification	Mass
Histology	131	59
Benign	89	45
Malignant	43 (33%)	13 (22%)

SCREENING FOR BREAST CANCER

The purpose of screening is to discover those among the apparently well who are suffering from a particular disease (Wilson and Jungner, 1968). When the cause of the disease is not known primary prevention is not possible, and secondary prevention, which is the detection of the disease at an early stage when treatment can be effective, becomes of paramount importance. Effective treatment is one of the keys to successful screening and the value of screening for malignant or other incurable diseases has been questioned (Whitby, 1968), particularly when the results of treatment of breast cancer do not appear to have changed significantly in the last three decades.

The continuing high incidence of breast cancer in Western society makes it the commonest cause of death from malignant disease in middle-aged women. The distressing symptoms of disseminated disease are such that many women and their doctors are prepared to seek early diagnosis and treatment in an effort to prevent death from breast cancer. The overall curability of breast cancer may be in doubt (Brinkley and Haybittle, 1975) but we do know that prolonged survival without evidence of widespread metastases is most commonly associated with the treatment of small tumours which are confined to the breast (Adair, 1974). In addition to the fear of disseminated disease or death, many women find it difficult to face the loss of a breast. There is increasing evidence from present day clinical studies that limited surgery combined with radiotherapy may allow conservation of the breast without a deterioration in the quality or duration of survival. This gives an added impetus to the need for early detection.

A randomized controlled clinical trial – the HIP study in New York – has already shown that screening for breast cancer by palpation and mammography can improve the survival of women over the age of 50 in the ten years of follow-up since the trial was completed (Shapiro, 1977).

The prognosis of breast cancer after diagnosis and primary treatment is related to a number of factors, among the most important of which are the size of the tumour and the histological status of the regional (axillary) lymph nodes (Bloom and Richardson, 1957; Bloom, 1965; Champion et al., 1972; Crile, 1972). Involvement of those nodes with metastatic tumour reduces survival (Fisher and Slack, 1970), but there is evidence to suggest that the addition of systemic therapy with hormones (Meakin et al., 1979) or cytotoxic chemotherapy (Bonadonna et al., 1977) can delay the onset of recurrence or metastatic disease or possibly prolong survival.

Attempts to improve diagnostic techniques in the last 15 years has shown that the standard procedures of palpation and mammography applied to women without symptoms have produced a yield of smaller or minimal tumours with a lower frequency of axillary lymph node involvement than is normally seen in women presenting at breast diagnostic clinics with symptoms (Davey et al., 1970; Stark and Way, 1974). When screening tests are used on women without symptoms the chance that evidence of disease will be found is low and it is necessary to screen large populations in order to detect even a small number of cancers. The costs and risks of doing this may be excessive and the problem is currently being attacked in two ways.

Population screening

The New York HIP study was a carefully designed randomized controlled clinical trial using physical examination and mammography, in which the incidence and results of treatment of breast cancer were recorded in a population that was identifiable and controlled by virtue of its investment in and association with an insurance plan (Strax et al., 1973). The details of the control population and the study population was such that the two groups were very comparable (Shapiro, 1977). The information gained from the study does not of course tell us anything about the incidence of breast cancer in the whole of metropolitan New York.

There are many methods of screening. Presently in Britain the National

Breast Cancer Screening Trial which is sponsored by the Department of Health and Social Security has the aim of studying breast cancer screening in populations of women aged between 35 and 65 in geographical areas. Screening by different techniques is being tested in four separate centres, the prevalence, incidence and survival of breast cancer patients is being recorded in these districts and compared with information obtained from four similar demographic areas which do not have the benefit of screening programmes (DHSS, 1981). In two of the centres, the screening techniques are of palpation and mammography and in two other centres, the technique is regular self-examination. All centres have standardized documentation and there is pathological collaboration between the histopathologists in each centre. Breast cancer is not one disease but a group of diseases and the importance of a careful and standardized histopathological control cannot be overemphasized (Azzopardi, 1979).

Such population screening programmes should record and analyse, amongst other factors, the age specific incidence and mortality rates, the epidemiological or risk factors that might affect the chances of developing breast cancer, the response of women to self-diagnosis, the effectiveness of the screening tests applied and the order and frequency in which those tests are used, the costs of the tests and the costs of further investigations including biopsy in those with true positive, false positive and true negative results. Other complicating factors will include the results of previous screening examinations and the possibility of delayed diagnosis of cancer through false negative results at screening. These are complex, interrelated problems and their analysis becomes more difficult with increasing numbers of screening tests.

In Sweden, Lundgren and Jakobsson have shown that a single test can be a worthwhile method of population screening (Lundgren and Jakobsson, 1976; Lundgren, 1977). Their project demonstrated that single oblique view mammography, on its own, was an effective and sensitive screening test in the detection of prevalent cancer at an initial examination and of incident cancer at subsequent examinations. Women examined by this technique were asked if they were aware of any lump in the breasts and when that information was combined with the information from the single radiograph of each breast it was possible to diagnose more than 90% of the cancers in that population of women. This method allowed palpation of the breast to be omitted from the screening procedure at the initial attendance. The results of their investigation showed that clinical examination of the breast in women with a normal mammogram and who were not aware of a lump in the breast themselves did not significantly contribute to breast cancer detection.

However, the costs of mass population screening are such that their general application is not justified when resources are limited until a proper cost benefit analysis has been made (*Lancet* Leading article, 1982; Miller and Bulbrook, 1982). Apart from the overt costs of the tests with the costs of labour and materials involved there are the unassessable psychological costs of false positive diagnoses with the anxiety associated with breast biopsy. Conversely it is difficult to assess the benefit of the reassurance given to an anxious woman by a negative physical examination and a negative mammogram.

High risk group screening

The selective use of screening techniques on women thought to be at high risk for developing breast cancer is an approach currently under investigation (Shapiro *et al.*, 1968; Egan, 1979). In considering who should be screened the age distribution and incidence of breast cancer are important in identifying those at greatest risk. The age specific incidence rate rises steadily with age but the age distribution of breast cancer peaks between the ages of 45 and 49 and is a plateau between the ages of 50 and 75. Apart from sex, age is the most important factor in the development of breast cancer, and screening programmes should probably not apply to women under the age of 40. A maternal family history of breast cancer doubles the risk of a particular patient developing the disease from about 1 in 15 to 1 in 8. The anxiety caused by such personal contact with the disease is considerable, even though viewed optimistically this must mean that the patient has 7 chances in 8 of not developing breast cancer. The studies at the MD Anderson Hospital in Houston (Anderson, 1971 and 1974) have shown that the daughters of mothers with breast cancer develop it approximately 10 years earlier and when mother and sister are both affected the risk increases fifty-fold.

The age at menarche and the age at menopause are both associated with varying risks of the development of breast cancer since it seems the disease is commoner in women who have an earlier menarche and a late menopause. It is also commoner in the unmarried and nulliparous (MacMahon *et al.*, 1973).

There are a number of reports that suggest an association between benign breast disease (benign mammary dysplasia, fibroadenosis, fibro-cystic disease, chronic cystic mastitis) and the detection of carcinoma. The pathological changes of benign mammary dysplasia are varied and they probably represent a spectrum of ageing in a gland which is stimulated in a cyclical way for 30–40 years of a woman's life. Certainly the symptoms of the disease, pain, lumpiness and occasionally the appearance of discrete masses, are prevalent in the reproductive life of many women. These symptoms lead to the patient seeking medical opinion which can lead to a significant biopsy rate and much of that surgery is carried out to exclude a diagnosis of malignant disease. This will usually be the case but in a number unsuspected tumours will be found, particularly of the *in situ* variety. In this way women with benign breast disease develop an increased chance of an occult carcinoma being discovered. Haagensen (1971) indicated a four-fold increase in the risk of developing breast cancer in women with such changes in their breasts. There seems little doubt that the significant histological feature of benign mammary dysplasia which predisposes to subsequent malignancy is epithelial hyperplasia, either within major or minor ducts or within the breast lobules (Davis, 1964, Foote, 1945, Gallager and Martin, 1969).

So far, data concerning the association of exogenous endocrine administration either in the contraceptive pill or in the form of hormone replacement therapy is inconclusive due to the lack of long-term follow-up of its usage in large population groups. Other possible aetiological factors include the smoking habits of the patient, the use of hair dye, their psychological make-up and even the high fat intake in the diet of affluent societies. At present the precise influence of these factors is not clear because of the lack of corroborative data.

Since 1968 we have developed an Early Diagnostic Breast Clinic at The Royal Marsden Hospital which has offered examinations to women with minimal symptoms. At the outset, women were self-referred and were examined clinically and thermographically; mammography being used only when there was a clinical or thermographic abnormality. This approach led to several biopsies and the detection of some cancers. Because of limited facilities we adopted a policy of seeing women referred from and by their family practitioners with minimal symptoms or for screening without symptoms. We continued to use thermography as an indicator of abnormality (and not as a diagnostic examination) and we used xeromammography increasingly as a routine method of examination of women aged 40 and over.

Table 11.2   Attendances at Early Diagnostic Clinic, Royal Marsden Hospital.

2 year periods	New cases	Re-attendances	Total
1968–69	2759	2740	5499
1972–73	1509	7033	8542
1974–75	866	5754	6620
1977–78	2301	16034	18335

Table 11.2 gives a summary of our experience in four separate periods, each of two years duration. The re-attendance figures result from further screening visits offered to women who have been found normal at the outset or who have been classified as having benign mammary dysplasia not requiring biopsy. Between 50–60% of women re-attend following an initial visit.

The abnormalities found in the screening clinics are reassessed by discussion between clinician and radiologist – reviewing the findings together and re-examining the women in a review clinic. The weekly review clinic leads to a surgical decision about the need for biopsy. Fine needle aspiration cytology has contributed significantly in the last five years to a reduction in the biopsy rate. This is shown in Table 11.3 and, in addition to the reduction in the biopsies in relation to the numbers of women seen, there has also been an improvement in the ratio of malignant

Table 11.3 Biopsies from Early Diagnostic Clinic.

2 year periods	Total	Benign	Cancer	Ratio of malignant:benign
1968–69	194	175	19	1:8
1972–73	240	204	36	1:6
1974–75	174	133	41	1:3
1977–78	142	104	38	1:2.5

to benign biopsies – one of our aims in the review clinic is to reduce the number of unnecessary benign biopsies. While it is easy for a surgeon to recommend a biopsy (to exclude malignancy) this causes considerable anxiety to the woman and it is an additional burden on the surgical facilities. In our own practice the largest proportion of benign biopsies still come from the firm, nodular, dysplastic breast in which mammography is not suspicious and from which fine needle aspiration has yielded benign cytology.

Thus the majority of women passing through a screening clinic of this kind are found to be normal and one of our prospective studies is an examination of the intervals needed to screen women for breast cancer. One of the important features of screening is the ability to examine women between routine appointments and the need to do this is generated by their own discovery of an abnormality in the breast, commonly a lump. Breast self-examination is thought to be an important part of the earlier detection of breast cancer and certainly most tumours are still found by women themselves. Unfortunately, not all women are willing to practise regular self-examination and indeed some find it a particularly frightening experience (Gray, 1981; Venet, 1980).

Conversely a minority of women in the screening clinic have some abnormality which requires surgical review and these may require an open biopsy to diagnose or exclude carcinoma. Of the first 105 carcinomas detected in this clinic, 50 were at the first visit ('prevalent'), 38 at a subsequent routine screen ('incident') and 17 were found by the women who asked for an early appointment ('interval'). Table 11.4 shows the clinical staging of these tumours and the majority are in Stage I or are non-infiltrating cancers. This is confirmed by the pathological staging of the

Table 11.4 Clinical stage of 105 cancers

	Non-invasive		Infiltrating	
	Total	*In situ*	Stage I	Stage II, III, IV
Asymptomatic	22	7	12	3
Symptomatic	83	10	57	16

Table 11.5   Pathological stage of 88 infiltrating carcinomas and axillary histology.

	Total	Negative	Positive	% negative
Asymptomatic	15	13	2	87
Symptomatic	73 (6 not known)	41	26	61

axilla and in Table 11.5 it is seen, from a small number of cases, that the detection of tumours – of which the patient herself was unaware – reduced the rate of axillary node invasion. This must improve the prognosis for those women with minimal, invasive breast carcinoma.

The continuing aims of such a clinic remain those which were posed at the beginning of this chapter. It is possible to detect minimal or early (low) stage carcinomas and if this is done before the onset of symptoms, the long term prognosis for individual women may be excellent. It will be important to evaluate the cost benefits of such a programme in relation to the diagnosis and treatment of 'early' or minimal breast carcinoma and relate this to the more extensive costs of diagnosis and treatment for advanced disease.

BIBLIOGRAPHY

AARTS, N.J.M. (1969) *Medische Thermographie*, Bergman, Tilberry, p. 38.

ABRAMSON, D.J. (1976) Delayed mastectomy after out-patient breast biopsy. Long-term survival study. *Am. J. Surg.*, **132**, 596.

ADAIR, F., BERG, J., JOUBERT, L. and ROBBINS, G. (1974) Long term follow-up of breast cancer patients. The 30 year report. *Cancer*, **33**, 1145–50.

AMALRIC, R., SPITALIER, J.M., LEVRAUD, J. and ALTSHULER, C. (1972) Les Images Thermovisuelles des Cancers du Sein et leur Classification. *Semin. AGA Thermovis. Cor. Médit. Med.*, **216**, 13–22.

AMALRIC, R., SPITALIER, J.M., GIRAUD, D. and ALTSHULER, C. (1975) Thermography in diagnosis of breast diseases. Thermogr. Proc. 1st. Europ. Congr., (Amsterdam 1974) *Bibl. Radiol.*, **6**, 65–76.

ANDERSEN, J.A. (1977) Lobular carcinoma *in situ*. A long-term follow-up in 52 cases. *Acta path. microbiol. scand.*, sect. A.82, 519–33.

ANDERSEN, J.A. (1977) Lobular carcinoma *in situ* of the breast. An approach to rational treatment. *Cancer*, **39**, 2597–602.

ANDERSON, D. (1971) Some characteristics of familial breast cancer. *Cancer*, **28**, 1500–4.

ANDERSON, D. (1974) Genetic study of breast cancer: identification of a high risk group. *Cancer*, **34**, 1090–7.

ANDERSON, J.M. (1980) Inflammatory carcinomas of the breast. *Ann. R. Coll. Surg.*, **62**, 195–9.

ANDERSSON, I., HILDELL, J., MUHLOW, A. and PETTERSSON, H. (1978) Number of projections in mammography: influence on detection of breast disease. *Am. J. Roentgenol.*, **130**, 349–51.

ANDERSSON, I., ANDREN, L., HILDELL, J., LINELL, F. *et al.* (1979) Breast Cancer screening with mammography. *Radiology*, **132**, 273–6.

ARNOLD, B.A., WEBSTER, E.W., and KALISHER, L. (1978) Evaluation of mammographic screen-film systems. *Radiology*, **129**, 179–85.

ARNOLD, B.A., EISENBERG, H. and BJÄRNGARD, B.E. (1979) Magnification mammography: a low dose technique. *Radiology*, **131**, 743–9.

ARTHES, G.G., SALTWELL, P.E. and LEWISON, E. (1971) The pill, estrogens and the breast. *Cancer*, **28**, 1391.

ASHIKARI, R., HUVOS, A.G., URBAN, J.A. and ROBBINS, G.F. (1973) Infiltrating lobular carcinoma of the breast. *Cancer*, **31**, 110–16.

ATKINS, H.J.B. and WOLFF, B. (1964) Discharge from the nipple. *Br. J. Surg.*, **51**, 602–6.

ATTIYEH, F.F., JENSEN, M., HUVOS, A.G. and FRACCHIA, A. (1977) Axillary micrometastasis and macrometastasis in carcinoma of the breast. *Surg. Gynaec. Obstet.*, **144**, 839–42.

AZZOPARDI, J.G. (1979) In *Problems in Breast Pathology. Major problems in Pathology 11.* (ed. J.L. Bennington), W.B. Saunders Company Ltd, London, Philadelphia, Toronto, pp. 23–5 (a); pp. 92–112 (b); pp. 183–4 (c).

BAILAR, J.C. (1976) Mammography – a contrary view. *Ann. Intern. Med.*, **84**, 77–84.

BARNES, G.T. and BREZOVICH, I.A. (1978) The intensity of scattered radiation in mammography. *Radiology*, **126**, 243–7.

BARRETT, A.H., MYERS, P.C. and SADOWSKY, N.L. (1980) Microwave thermography in the detection of breast cancer. *Am. J. Roentgenol.*, **134**, 365–8.

BASSETT, L.W., GOLD, R.H. and COVE, H.C. (1978) Mammographic spectrum of traumatic fat necrosis: the fallibility of 'pathognomonic' signs of carcinoma. *Am. J. Roentgenol.*, **130**, 119–22.

BECKER, W. (1979) Stereotactic localization of breast lesions. *Radiology*, **133**, 238–40.

B.E.N.T. (1978) *Breast Exposure: nationwide trends. A mammographic quality assurance programme.* U.S. Department of Health, Education and Welfare. Bureau of Radiological Health, Rockville, Maryland.

BERG, J.W. (1955) The significance of axillary node levels in the study of breast carcinoma. *Cancer*, **8**, 776–8.

BETSILL, W.L., ROSEN, P.P., LEIBERMAN, P.H. and ROBBINS, G.F. (1978) Intraductal carcinoma. Long-term follow-up after treatment by biopsy alone. *J. Am. Med. Assoc.*, **239**, 1863–7.

BIRNBAUM, S.F. (1966) Breast temperature as a test for pregnancy. *Obstet. Gynaecol. NY*, **27**, 378–80.

BJORN-HANSEN, R. (1965) Contrast mammography. *Br. J. Radiol.*, **38**, 947–51.

BLACK, M.M., BARCLAY, T.H.C. and HANKEY, B.F. (1975) Prognosis in breast cancer utilising histologic characteristics of the primary tumour. *Cancer*, **36**, 2048–55.

BLACK, M.M., OPLER, S.R. and SPEER, F.D. (1955) Survival in breast cancer cases in relation to the structure of the primary tumour and regional lymph nodes. *Surg. Gynaecol. Obstet.*, **100**, 543–51.

BLACK, M.M., SPEER, F.D. and OPLER, S.R. (1956) Structural representations of tumour-host relationships in mammary carcinoma. Biologic and prognostic significance. *Am. J. Clin. Path.*, **26**, 250–65.

BLOOM, H.J.G. and RICHARDSON, W.W. (1957) Histological grading and prognosis in breast cancer. *Br. J. Cancer*, **11**, 359–77.

BLOOM, H.J.G. (1965) The influence of delay on the natural history and prognosis of breast cancer. *Br. J. Cancer*, **19**, 228.

BOAG, J.W. (1973a) Xeroradiography. *Physics Med. Biol.*, **18**, 3–37.

BOAG, J.W. (1973b) in *Modern Trends in Oncology 1, Part two: clinical progress* (Ed. R.W. Raven), Butterworths, London, pp. 79–89.

BOAG, J.W. (1975) in *Biomedical Dosimetry*, I.A.E.A., Vienna, pp. 475–98.

BONADONNA, G., ROSSI, A., VALAGUSSA, P., BANFI, A. and VERONESI, U. (1977) The CMF program of operable breast cancer with positive axillary nodes: updated analysis on the disease-free interval, site of relapse and drug tolerance. *Cancer*, **39**, 2904–15.

BRINKLEY, D. and HAYBITTLE, J.L. (1975) The curability of breast cancer. *Lancet*, **ii**, 95.

BRODY, E. (1980) Cancer Society reports it finds some detection tests unneeded. *New York Times.*

BROWN, P.W., SILVERMAN, J., OWENS, E., TABOR, D.C. *et al.* (1976) Intraductal 'non-infiltrating' carcinoma of the breast. *Arch. Surg.*, 3, 1063–7.

BUCANOSSI, P. and VERONESI, U. (1957) Some observations of cancer of the breast in mothers and daughters. *Br. J. Cancer*, 3, 337.

BUCHANAN, J.B. and JAGER, R.M. (1977) Single view negative mode xeromammography. An approach to reduce radiation exposure in breast cancer screening. *Radiology*, 123, 63–8.

BULBROOK, R.D., HAYWARD, J. and SPICER, C. (1971) Relation between urinary androgen and corticoid excretion and subsequent breast cancer. *Lancet*, ii, 395–8.

BUSK, T. and CLEMMESON, J. (1947) Frequencies of left and right sided breast cancer. *Br. J. Cancer*, 1, 345.

BYRNE, R.R. and YERES, J.A. (1975) The three roles of breast thermography. *Appl. Radiol.*, 4, 53–8.

CARPENTER, D., KOSSOFF, G., CARRETT, W.J., DANIEL, K. and BOELE, P. (1977) The U.I. Octoson – a new class of ultrasonic echoscope. *Australas. Radiol.*, 21, 85–9.

CARROLL, K.K. (1975) Experimental evidence of dietary factors and hormone-dependent carcinomas. *Cancer Res.*, 35, 3374.

CHAMBERLAIN, J. (1975) The feasibility of clinical and radiological screening for breast neoplasm. *Proc. R. Soc. Med.*, 68, 431.

CHAMPION, H.R., WALLACE, I.W.J. and PRESCOTT, R.J. (1972) Histology in breast cancer prognosis. *Br. J. Cancer*, 26, 129–38.

CHANG, C.H.J., SIBALA, J.L., MARTIN, N.L. and RILEY, R.C. (1976) Film mammography: new low radiation technology. *Radiology*, 121, 215–17.

CLARK, R.M., RIDEOUT, D.F. and CHART, P.L. (1978) Thermography of the breast: experiences in diagnosis and follow-up in a cancer treatment centre. *Acta thermogr.*, 3, 155–61.

COOMBS, L.J., LILIENFELD, A.M., BROSS, I.D.J. and BURNETT, W.S. (1979) A prospective study of the relationship between benign breast disease and breast carcinoma. *Prev. Med.*, 8, 40–52.

CRILE, G. (1972) Breast cancer: relationship of the size of tumour and the size of involved nodes to survival. *Am. J. Surg.*, 124, 35–8.

CROLL, J. (1980) '*You need to put more than a finger on the breasts these days*'. Abstract 260, Combined Meeting of Royal Australasian College of Surgeons, Royal Australasian College of Physicians and Royal College of Physicians and Surgeons of Canada, Sydney, Australia. (February).

CUBILLA, A.L. and WOODRUFF, J.M. (1977) Primary carcinoid tumour of the breast. A report of eight patients. *Am. J. Surg. Path.*, 1, 283–92.

CUTLER, S.J., ZIPPIN, C. and ASIRE, A.J. (1969) The prognostic significance of palpable lymph nodes in cancer of the breast. *Cancer*, 23, 243.

DANCE, D.R. (1980) The Monte Carlo calculation of integral radiation dose in xeromammography. *Physics Med. Biol.*, 25, 25–37.

DANCE, D.R. and DAY, G.J. (1981) Simulation of mammography by Monte Carlo Calculation – the dependence of radiation dose, scatter and noise on photon energy in *Proceedings of Patient Exposure to Radiation in Medical X-ray Diagnosis*, Munich 1981 (eds G. Drexler, H. Eriskat and H. Schibilla), CEC, Luxembourg, pp. 227–43, EUR 7438.

DAVEY, J.B., MCKINNA, J.A. and GREENING, W.P. (1970) Is screening for cancer worthwhile? Results from a well-woman clinic for cancer detection. *Br. Med. J.*, **3**, 696–9.

DAVIS, H.H., SIMONS, M. and DAVIS, J.B. (1964) Cystic disease of the breast: relationship to carcinoma. *Cancer*, **17**, 957–78.

DAVIS, R., DANCE, D.R., PARSONS, C.A. and BAKER, A.M. (1980) The reduction of dose in xeromammography by the use of aluminium filters (unpublished).

DAVISON, T.W., EQING, K.L., FERGASON, J., CHAPMAN, M. *et al.* (1972) Detection of breast cancer by liquid crystal thermography. *Cancer*, **29**, 1123–32.

DENOIX, P. (1970) *Treatment of Malignant Breast Tumours (Recent Results in Cancer Research*, vol. 31) William Heinemann Medical Books Ltd, London, pp. 6–11.

DE WAARD, F. (1975) Breast cancer incidence and nutritional status with particular reference to body weight and height. *Cancer. Res.*, **35**, 3351.

DE WERD, L.A. (1979) *Quality assurance in mammography – diagnosis of artefact sources in xeroradiographic systems*. N.I.H. publication 79 – 1684. U.S. Department of Health, Education and Welfare.

DHSS WORKING GROUP (1981) Trial of early detection of breast cancer: description of method. *Br. J. Cancer*, **44**, 618–27.

DODD, G.D., WALLACE, J.D., FREUNDLICH, I.M., MARSH, L. and ZERMEND, A. (1969) Thermography and cancer of the breast. *Cancer*, **23**, 797–802.

DODD, G.D. (1977) Present status of thermography, ultrasound and mammography in breast cancer detection. *Cancer*, **39**, 2796–805.

DRAPER, J.W. and JONES, C.H. (1969) Thermal patterns of the female breast. *Br. J. Radiol.*, **42**, 401–10.

DRAPER, J.W. and BOAG, J.W. (1971) Skin temperature distribution over veins and tumours. *Physics Med. Biol.*, **16**, 645–54.

DUBUQUE, G.L., CACAK, R.K. and HENDEE, W.R. (1977) Backscatter factors in the mammographic energy range. *Med. Physics*, **4**, 397–9.

DUGUID, H.L.D., WOOD, R.A.B., IRVING, A.D., PREECE, P.E. and CUSCHIERI, A. (1979) Needle aspiration of the breast with immediate reporting of material. *Br. Med. J.*, **2**, 185.

EDRICH, J. (1978) *Microwave and millimeter wave thermography*. Abstract 14, European Congress of Thermography, Barcelona.

EGAN, R. (1979) Estimated risk and occurrence of breast cancer in asymptomatic and minimally symptomatic patients. *Cancer*, **43**, 871–7.

EGAN, R.L. and MCSWEENEY, M.B. (1979) Mammographic parenchymal patterns and risk of breast cancer. *Radiology*, **133**, 65–70.

EGELI, R.A. and URBAN, J.A. (1979) Mammography in symptomatic women 50 years of age and under and those over 50. *Cancer*, **43**, 878–82.

ELSTON, C.W., COTTON, R.E., DAVIES, C.J. and BLAMEY, R.W. (1978) A comparison of the use of the 'tru-cut' needle and fine needle aspiration cytology in the pre-operative diagnosis of carcinoma of the breast. *Histopath.*, **2**, 239–54.

ERDREICH, L.A., ASAL, N.R. and HOGE, A.F. (1980) Morphologic type of breast cancer. Age, bilaterality and family history. *South. Med. J.*, **73**, 26–32.

ERNSTER, V.L., SACKS, S.T., PETERSON, C.A. and SCHWEITZER, R.J. (1980) Mammographic parenchymal patterns and risk factors for breast cancer. *Radiology*, **134**, 617–20.

EUSEBI, V., BETTS, C.M. and BUSSOLATI, G. (1979) Tubular carcinoma: a variant of secretory breast carcinoma. *Histopath.*, **3**, 407–19.

EVANS, A.L., JAMES, W.B., MCLELLAN, J. and DAVIDSON, M. (1975) Film and xeroradiographic images in mammography. A comparison of tungsten and molybdenum anode materials. *Br. J. Radiol.*, **48**, 968–72.

FASAL, E. (1975) Oral contraceptives as related to cancer and benign lesions of the breast. *J. Natl. Cancer Inst.*, **55**, 767.

FEIG, S.A., LIBSHITZ, H.I. and SCHWARTZ, G.S. (1977) In *Breast Carcinoma: Radiologist's Expanded Role* (ed. W.W. Logan), Wiley Publishers, New York.

FEIG, S.A., SHABER, G.S., SCHWARTZ, G.F., PATCHEFSKY, A. *et al.* (1977) Thermography, mammography and clinical examination in breast cancer screening. *Radiology*, **122**, 123–7.

FENDER, W.D. (1975) Quantification of the xeroradiographic discharge curve. *Proc. Soc. Photo-Optical Instrumentation Engineers*, **70**, 364–71.

FENTIMAN, I.S., MILLIS, R.R. and HAYWARD, J.L. (1980) Value of needle biopsy in outpatient diagnosis of breast cancer. *Arch. Surg.*, **115**, 652–3.

FEWELL, T.R. and SHUPING, R.E. (1979) *Handbook of mammographic X-ray spectra.* H.E.W. Publication (FDA) 79, 8071. U.S. Department of Health, Education and Welfare.

FINK, R. (1976) *Delay behaviour in breast cancer screening: Cancer: the behavioural dimensions* (eds J.W. Cullen, B.H. Fox and R.N. Isom), Raven Press, New York

FISHER, B., RAVDIN, R.G., AUSMAN, R.K., SLACK, N.H. *et al.* (1968) Surgical adjuvant chemotherapy in cancer of the breast: results of a decade of cooperative investigation. *Ann. Surg.*, **168**, 337–56.

FISHER, B. and SLACK, N.H. (1970) Number of lymph nodes examined and the prognosis of breast carcinoma. *Surg. Gynaecol. Obstet.*, **131**, no. 1, 79–88.

FISHER, E.R., GREGORIO, R.M., REDMOND, C., KIM, W.S. and FISHER, B. (1976) Pathologic findings from the National Surgical Adjuvant Breast Project (Protocol no. 4) III. The significance of extranodal extension of axillary metastases. *Am. J. Clin. Path.*, **65**, 439–44.

FISHER, E.R. (1978) The pathologist's role in the diagnosis and treatment of invasive breast cancer. *Surg. Clin. N. Am.*, **58**, 705–21.

FISHER, E.R., PALEKAR, A., ROCKETTE, H., REDMOND, C. and FISHER, B. (1978) Pathological findings from the National Surgical Adjuvant Breast Project (Protocol no. 4) V. Significance of axillary nodal micro- and macrometastases. *Cancer*, **42**, 2032–8.

FISHER, E.R., SWAMIDOSS, S., LEE, C.H., ROCKETTE, H. *et al.* (1978) Detection and significance of occult axillary node metastases in patients with invasive breast cancer. *Cancer*, **42**, 2025–31.

FISHER, E.R., PALEKAR, A.S. and NSABP collaborators (1979) Solid and mucinous varieties of so-called mammary carcinoid tumours. *Am. J. Clin. Path.*, **72**, 909–16.

FITZGERALD, M., WHITE, D.R., WHITE, E. and YOUNG, J. (1979) *Mammography – current practice and dosimetry in Britain* (preprint), St. Bartholomew's Hospital, London.

FOOTE, F.W. and STEWART, F.W. (1941) Lobular carcinoma *in situ*. A rare form of mammary cancer. *Am. J. Path.*, **17**, 491–7.

FOOTE, F.W. and STEWART, F.W. (1945) Comparative studies of cancerous versus non-cancerous breasts. *Ann. Surg.*, **121**, 6–53, 197–222.

FORREST, H.P. (1966) Intraduct papilloma. *Br. J. Surg.*, **53**, 1028–32.

FOSTER, J., LANG, S., COSTANZA, M., WORDEN, J. *et al.* (1978) Breast self-examination practices and breast cancer stage. *New Engl. J. Med.*, **299**, (6), 265–70.

FOX, C. (1979) Innovation in medical diagnosis. The Scandinavian curiosity. *Lancet*, **i**, 1387–8.

FRANK, H.A., HALL, F.M. and STEER, M.L. (1976) Pre-operative localization of non-palpable breast lesions demonstrated by mammography. *New Engl. J. Med.*, **295**, 5, 259–60.

FRANKL, G. and ROSENFELD, D.D. (1973) Breast xeroradiography: analysis of our first seventeen months. *Ann. Surg.*, **178**, 676–9.

FREUNDLICH, I.M., WALLACE, J.D. and DODD, G.D. (1968) Thermography and the venous diameter ratio in the detection of non-palpable breast carcinoma. *Am. J. Roentgenol.*, **102**, 927–32.

FRIEDRICH, M. and WESKAMP, P. (1978) New modalities in mammographic imaging comparison of grid and magnification techniques. *Medicamundi*, **23**, 29–46.

FUNDERBURK, W.W. and SYPHAX, B. (1969) Evaluation of nipple discharge in benign and malignant diseases. *Cancer*, **24**, 1290–6.

FUNDERBURK, W.W., SYPHAX, B. and SMITH, C.W. (1964) Contrast mammography in breast discharge. *Surg. Gynaec. Obstet.*, **119**, 276–80.

GALLAGER, H.S. and MARTIN, J.E. (1969) Early phases in the development of breast cancer. *Cancer*, **24**, 1170.

GALLAGER, H.S. and MARTIN, J.E. (1971) An orientation to the concept of minimal breast cancer. *Cancer*, **28**, 1505–7.

GALLAGER, H.S. (1975) Breast specimen radiography. Obligatory, adjuvant and investigative. *Am. J. Clin. Path.*, **64**, 749–55.

GAUTHERIE, M. and GROS, C.M. (1976) Contribution of infra-red thermography to early diagnosis, pretherapeutic prognosis and postirradiation follow-up of breast carcinomas. *Medicamundi*, **21**, (3), 135–49.

GAJEWSKI, H. (1977) in *Mammography* (eds W. Hoeffken and M. Lanyi), George Thieme, Stuttgart, pp. 4–24.

GEORGE, W.D., GLEAVE, E.N., ENGLAND, P.C., WILSON, M.C. *et al.* (1976) Screening for Breast Cancer. *Br. Med. J.*, **2**, 858–60.

GEORGE, W.D., SELLWOOD, R.A., ASBURY, D. and HARTLEY, G. (1980) Role of non-medical staff in screening for breast cancer. *Br. Med. J.*, **1**, 147–9.

GERDEKI, T.I.M., HOGBIN, B.M., MELCHER, D.H. and SMITH, R.S. (1980) Aspiration cytology in pre-operative diagnosis of breast cancer. *Lancet*, **ii**, 790–2.

GERSHON-COHEN, J. (1970) *Atlas of Mammography*, Springer Verlag, Berlin, Heidelberg, New York.

GILERSKUPPER, B., URCA, I. and MOROZ, C. (1979) Immunodiagnostic test for the early detection of carcinoma of the breast. *Gynaecol. Obstet.*, **149**, (5), 655–6.

GOLINGER, R., CUR, D., FISHER, B., HERBERT, D. *et al.* (1979) The significance of concordance in mammographic interpretations. *Cancer*, **44**, 1252–5.

GRAVELLE, I.H., BULSTRODE, J.C., WANG, D.Y. and HAYWARD, J.L. (1980) The relation between radiographic features and determinants of risk of breast cancer. *Br. J. Radiol.*, **53**, 107–13.

GRAY, L.A. (1981) The role of breast self-examination in the detection of breast cancers. *Breast, Dis. Breast*, **7**, 6–8.

GREER, S. and MORRIS, T. (1975) Psychological attributes of women who develop breast cancer; a controlled study. *J. Psychosom. Res.*, **19**, 147–53.

GRIFFITHS, K. (1978) Ultrasound examination of the breast. *Med. Ultrasound.*, **2**, 13–19.

GROS, C.H., GAUTHERIE, M., BOURJAT, P. and VROUSOS, C. (1969) Les applications médicales de la thermographie infra-rouge. *Acta electron*, **12**, 63–119.

GRUBB, C. (1981) *Colour Atlas of Breast Cytopathology*, HM & M Publishers Ltd, London.

HAAGENSEN, C.D. (1971) *Disease of the Breast*, 2nd edn, W.B. Saunders and Co., Philadelphia.

HAAGENSEN, C.D., LANE, N., LATTES, R. and BODIAN, C. (1978) Lobular neoplasia (so-called lobular carcinoma *in situ*) of the breast. *Cancer*, **42**, 737–69.

HAMBLIN LETTON, A., WILSON, J. and MASON, E. (1977) The value of breast screening in women less than fifty years of age. *Cancer*, **40**, 1–3.

HAMLIN, I.M.E. (1968) Possible host resistance in carcinoma of the breast: a histological study. *Br. J. Cancer*, **XXII**, 383–401.

HAMMERSTEIN, G.R., MILLER, D.W., WHITE, D.R., MASTERSON, M.E. *et al.* (1979) Absorbed radiation dose in mammography. *Radiology*, **130**, 485–91.

HANDLEY, R.S. (1972) Observations and thoughts on cancer of the breast. *Proc. R. Soc. Med.*, **65**, 437.

HARRIS, M., WELLS, S. and VASUDEV, K.S. (1978) Primary signet ring cell carcinoma of the breast. *Histopathology.*, **2**, 171–6.

HAUS, A.G. (1977) in *Breast Carcinoma: the Radiologist's Expanded Role* (ed. W.W. Logan), John Wiley and Sons Inc., New York, pp. 93–107.

HAUS, A.G., DOI, K., METZ, C.E. and BERNSTEIN, J. (1977) Image quality in mammography. *Radiology*, **125**, 77–85.

HAUS, A.G., METZ, C.E., CHILES, J.T. and ROSSMAN, K. (1976) The effect of X-ray spectra from molybdenum and tungsten target tubes on image quality in mammography. *Radiology*, **118**, 705–9.

HESSLER, C., SCHNYDER, P. and OZZELLO, L. (1978) Hamartoma of the breast: diagnostic observation of 16 cases. *Radiology*, **126**, 95–8.

HEUSER, L., SPRATT, J.S. and POLK, H.C. (1979) Growth rates of primary breast cancers. *Cancer*, **43**, 1888–94.

HEUSER, L., SPRATT, J.S., POLK, H.C. and BUCHANAN, J. (1979) Relation between mammary cancer growth kinetics and the intervals between screenings. *Cancer*, **43**, 857–62.

HICKEN, N.F. (1937) Mammography: roentgenographic diagnosis of breast tumours by means of contrast media. *Surg., Gynaec. Obstet.*, **64**, 593–603.

HICKEN, N.F., BEST, R.R., HUNT, H.B. and HARRIS, T.T. (1938) Roentgen visualization and diagnosis of breast lesions by means of contrast medium. *Am. J. Roentgenol.*, **39**, 321–43.

HOEFFKEN, W. and LANYI, M. (1977) *Mammography*, W.B. Saunders Co., Philadelphia, London, Toronto; George Thieme Publishers, Stuttgart.

HOFFMAN, R.L. (1967) Thermography in the detection of breast malignancy. *Am. J. Obstet. Gynaecol.*, **98**, 681–4.

HOOVER, R., GRAY, L., COLE, P. and MACMAHON, B. (1976) Menopausal estrogens and breast cancer. *New Engl. J. Med.*, **295**, 8, 401–5.

HORNS, J.W. and ARNDT, R.D. (1976) Percutaneous spot localization of non-palpable breast lesions. *Am. J. Roentgenol.*, **127**, 253–6.

HULL, M.T., SEO, I.S., BATTERSBY, J.S. and CSICSKO, J.F. (1980) Signet ring cell carcinoma of the breast: a clinicopathologic study of 24 cases. *Am. J. Clin. Path.*, **73**, 31–5.

HUTCHINSON, W.B., THOMAS, D.B., HAMLIN, W.B., ROTH, G.J. *et al.* (1980) Risk of breast cancer in women with benign breast diseases. *J. Natl. Cancer Inst.*, **65**, 13–20.

HUTTER, R.V.P., SNYDER, R.E., LUCAS, J.C., FOOT, F.W. and FARROW, J.H. (1969) Clinical and pathological correlation with mammographic findings in lobular carcinoma *in situ*. *Cancer*, **23**, 826–39.

HUVOS, A.G., HUTTER, R.V.P. and BERG, J.W. (1971) Significance of axillary macrometastases and micrometastases in mammary cancer. *Ann. Surg.*, **173**, 44–6.

HUVOS, A.G., LUCAS, L.C. and FOOTE, F.W. (1973) Metaplastic breast carcinoma: rare form of mammary cancer. *NY State J. Med.*, **73**, 1078–82.

I.C.R.P. Publication 15. (1970) *Protection against ionising radiation from external sources*, Pergamon Press, Oxford, p. 10.

ING, R., HO, J.H.C. and PETRAKIS, N.L. (1977) Unilateral breast-feeding and breast cancer. *Lancet*, **ii**, 124–7.

ISARD, H.J., BECKER, W., SHILO, R. and OSTRUM, B.J. (1972) Breast thermography after four years and 10 000 studies. *Am. J. Roentgenol.*, **115**, 811–21.

ISARD, H.J. (1972) Thermographic 'edge sign' in breast carcinoma. *Cancer*, **30**, 957–63.

JANS, R.G., BUTLER, P.F., MCCROHAN, J.L. and THOMPSON, W.E. (1979) The status of film/screen mammography. *Radiology*, **132**, 197–200.

JELLINS, J., KOSSOFF, G.W., BUDDEE, F.W. and REEVE, T.S. (1971) Ultrasonic visualization of the breast. *Med. J. Aust.*, **1**, 305–7.

JELLINS, J., KOSSOFF, G., REEVE, T.S. and BARRACLOUGH, B.H. (1975a) Ultrasonic grey scale visualization of breast disease. *Ultrasound Med. Biol.*, **1**, 393–404.

JELLINS, J., KOSSOFF, G. and REEVE, T.S. (1975b) The ultrasonic appearance of pathology in the male breast. *Ultrasound Med. Biol.*, **2**, 43–4.

JELLINS, J., KOSSOFF, G. and REEVE, T.S. (1977) Detection and classification of liquid filled masses in the breast by grey scale echography. *Radiology*, **125**, 205–12.

JELLINS, J., REEVE, T.S., CROLL, J. and KOSSOFF, G. (1982) Results of breast echographic examinations in Sydney, Australia, 1972–79. *Semin. Ultrasound*, **Vol. III**, No. 1.

JOHANSSON, N.T., BJÜRSTAM, N., HEDBERG, K., HULTBORN, A. and JOHNSEN, C. (1976) Thermography of the breast. *Acta chir. Scand, Supp.*, 460.

JONES, C.H. (1982) Methods of breast imaging. *Phys. Med. Biol.*, **27**, 463–99.

JONES, C.H. and DRAPER, J.W. (1970) A comparison of infra-red photography and thermography in the detection of mammary carcinoma. *Br. J. Radiol.*, **43**, 507–16.

JONES, C.H., GREENING, W.P., DAVEY, J.B., MCKINNA, J.A. and GREEVES, V.J. (1975) Thermography of the female breast: a five-year study in relation to the detection and prognosis of cancer. *Br. J. Radiol.*, **48**, 532–8.

KALISHER, L. (1979) Factors influencing false negative rates in xeromammography. *Radiology*, **133**, 297–301.

KISTER, S.J., SOMMERS, S.C., HAAGENSEN, C.D., FRIEDELL, G.H. *et al.* (1969) Nuclear grade and sinus histiocytosis in cancer of the breast. *Cancer*, **23**, 570–5.

KOBAYASHI, T. (1978) *Clinical ultrasound of the breast*, Plenum Medical Book Co, New York, p. 110.

KOSSOFF, G., GARRETT, W.J., CARPENTER, D.A., JELLINS, J. and DADD, M.J. (1976) Principals and classification of soft tissue by grey scale echography. *Ultrasound Med. Biol.*, **2**, 89–105.

KOSSOFF, G., JELLINS, J. and REEVE, T.S. (1978) in *Cancer Campaign* (vol, 1), Gustav Fischer Verlag, Stuttgart, pp. 149–58.

KREUZER, G. (1978) Aspiration biopsy cytology in proliferating benign mammary dysplasia. *Acta Cytol.*, **22**, (3), 128–32.

LAPAYOWKER, M.S., KUNDEL, H.L. and ZISKIN, M. (1971) Thermographic patterns of the female breast and their relationship to carcinoma. *Cancer*, **27**, 819–22.

LEADING ARTICLE (1978) Screening for breast cancer. Report from Edinburgh Breast Screening Clinic. *Br. Med. J.*, **2**, 175–8.

LEADING ARTICLE (1978) Screening for breast cancer. Statement by British Breast Group. *Br. Med. J.*, **2**, 178–80.

LEADING ARTICLE (1978) Back-up for screening for breast cancer. *Br. Med. J.*, **2**, 153–4.

LEADING ARTICLE (1979) Age and death in breast cancer. *Br. Med. J.*, **1**, 211–12.

LEADING ARTICLE (1982) Screening for breast cancer. *Lancet*, **i**, 1103.

LEBORGNE, R, (1951) Diagnosis of tumours of the breast by simple roentgenography. *Am. J. Roentgenol.*, **65**, 1.

LEWIS, J., MILBRATH, J., SHAFFER, K., DARIN, J. and DECOSSE, J. (1976) Which breast to biopsy? *Am. J. Surg.*, **184**, 253–6.

LIBSHITZ, H.I., FETOUH, S., ISLEY, J. and LESTER, R.G. (1976) One-view mammographic screening? *Radiology*, **120**, 719–22.

LILIENFELD, A.M., BARNES, J.M., BARNES, R.B., BRASFIELD, R. *et al.* (1969) An evaluation of thermography in the detection of breast cancer. *Cancer*, **24**, 1206–11.

LINELL, R., OSTBERG, G., SONDERSTROM, J., ANDERSSON, I. *et al.* (1979) Breast hamartomas: an important entity in mammary pathology. *Virchows Arch. Path. Anat. Histol.*, **383**, 253–64.

LOWE, C.R. and MacMAHON, B. (1970) Breast cancer and reproductive history of women in South Wales. *Lancet*, **i**, 153.

LUNDGREN, B. and JAKOBSSON, S. (1976) Single view mammography. *Cancer*, **38**, 1124–9.

LUNDGREN, B. (1977) The oblique view in mammography. *Br. J. Radiol.*, **50**, 626–8.

LUNDGREN, B. (1978) Malignant features of breast tumours at radiography. *Acta Radiol. Diagn.*, **19**, 623–33.

MacMAHON, B., COLE, P. and BROWN, J. (1973) Etiology of human breast cancer. A review. *J. Natl. Cancer Inst.*, **50**, 21.

MAMBO, N.C. and GALLAGER, H.S. (1977) Carcinoma of the breast. The prognostic significance of extranodal extension of axillary disease. *Cancer*, **39**, 2280–5.

MARSHALL, M., PEAPLE, L.H.J., ARDRAN, G.M. and CROOKS, H.E. (1975) A comparison of X-ray spectra and outputs from molybdenum and tungsten targets. *Br. J. Radiol.*, **48**, 31–9.

MARTIN, J.E. and GALLAGER, H.S. (1971) Mammographic diagnosis of minimal breast cancer. *Cancer*, **28**, 1519–26.

MARTINEZ, V. and AZZOPARDI, J.G. (1979) Invasive lobular carcinoma of the breast: incidence and variants. *Histopathology*, **3**, 467–88.

MASSOPUST, L.C. and GARDNER, W.D. (1953) The infra-red phlebogram in the diagnosis of breast complaints; analysis of 1 200 cases. *Surg. Gynaecol. Obstet.*, **97**, 619–26.

MCDIVITT, R.W., HUTTER, R.V.P., FOOTE, F.W. and STEWART, F.W. (1967) *In situ* lobular carcinoma. *JAMA*, **201**, 96–100.

MCDIVITT, R.W. (1978), Breast carcinoma. *Hum. Path.*, **9**, 3–21.

MCKINTOSH, I.H., HOOPER, A.A., MILLIS, R.R. and GREENING, W.P. (1976) Metastatic carcinoma within the breast. *Clin. Oncol.*, **2**, 393–401.

MEAKIN, J.W., ALT, W.E.C., BEALE, F.A., BROWN *et al.* (1979) Ovarian irradiation and prednisone therapy following surgery and radiotherapy for carcinoma of the breast. *Can. Med. Ass. J.*, **120**, 1221.

MILLER, A.B. and BULBROOK, R.D. (1982) Screening, detection and diagnosis of breast cancer. *Lancet*, i, 1109–11.

MILLIS, R.R., DAVIS, R. and STACEY, A.J. (1976) The detection and significance of calcifications in the breast: a radiological and pathological study. *Br. J. Radiol.*, **49**, 12–26.

MILLIS, R.R., GREENING, L.P. and MCKINNA, J.A. (1976b) Biopsy of the impalpable breast lesion detected by mammography. *Br. J. Surg.*, **63**, 346–8.

MILLIS, R.R. and THYNNE, G.S. (1975) *In situ* intraduct carcinoma of the breast; A long term follow up study. *Br. J. Surg.*, **62**, 957.

MINAGI, H. and YOUKER, J.E. (1968) Roentgen appearance of fat necrosis in the breast. *Radiology*, **90**, 62–5.

MINASIAN, H. and BAMBER, J.C. (1982) A preliminary assessment of an ultrasonic Doppler method for the study of blood flow in human breast cancer. *Ultrasound Med. Biol.*, **8**, (4), 357–64.

MOORES, B.M. (1980) *Review of physical assessment of image quality*. Paper presented at Symposium Mammographicum 1980, University College, London (5–6 September).

MOORES, B.M., HUFTON, A.P., WRIGLEY, C., ASBURY, D.L. and RAMSDEN, J.A. (1979) A quantitative evaluation of film and film/screen combinations for mammographic examination. *Br. J. Radiol.*, **52**, 626–33.

MOORES, B.M., RAMSDEN, J.A. and ASBURY, D.L. (1980) An atmospheric pressure ionographic system suitable for mammography. *Physics Med, Biol.*, **25**, 893–902.

MOSKOWITZ, M., PEMMARAJU, S., FIDLER, J., SUTORIUS, D. *et al.* (1976) On the diagnosis of minimal breast cancer in a screening population. *Cancer*, **37**, 2543–52.

MUELLER, C.B. and AMES, P. (1978) Bilateral carcinoma of the breast: frequency and mortality. *Can. J. Surg.*, **21**, 459–65.

MÜHLOW, A. (1974) A device for precision needle biopsy of the breast at mammography. *Am. J. Roentgenol.* **121**, No 4, 843–5.

NASCA, P.C., LAWRENCE, C.E., GREENWALD, P., CHORDST, S. *et al.* (1980) Relationship of hair dye use, benign breast disease and breast cancer. *J. Natl. Cancer Inst.*, **64**, 23–8.

NORDENSTROM, B. and ZAJICEK, J. (1977) Stereotaxic needle biopsy and pre-operative indication of non-palpable mammary lesions. *Acta Cytol.*, **21** (2), 350–1.

NORRIS, H.J. and TAYLOR, H.B. (1970) Carcinoma of the breast in women less than thirty years old. *Cancer*, **26**, 953–9.

OBERMAN, H.A. (1980) Secretory carcinoma of the breast in adults. *Am. J. Surg. Path.*, **4**, 465–70.

OSTRUM, B.J., BECKER, W. and ISARD, H.J. (1973) Low dose mammography. *Radiology*, **109**, 323–6.

OZZELLO, L. (1971) Ultrastructure of intra-epithelial carcinoma of the breast. *Cancer*, **28**, 1508–15.

PAGE, D.L., ZWAAG, R.V., ROGERS, L.W., WILLIAMS, L.T. *et al.* (1978) Relation between component parts of fibrocystic disease complex and breast cancer. *J. Natl. Cancer Inst.*, **61**, 1055–63.

PATCHEFSKY, A.S., SHABER, G.S., SCHWARTZ, G.F., FEIG, S.A. and NERLINGER, R.E. (1977) The pathology of breast cancer detected by mass population screening. *Cancer*, **40**, 1659–70.

PATEY, D.A. and SCARFF, R.W. (1928) Position of histology in prognosis of carcinoma of breast. *Lancet*, **i**, 801.

PAYNE, R.A. and JACKSON, D.B. (1980) Cystic tumours of the breast. *Ann. R. Coll. Surg.*, **62**, 228–9.

PETERS, M.V. (1968) The effect of pregnancy in breast cancer in *Prognostic Factors in Breast Cancer* (eds A.P.M. Forrest and P.B. Kunkler), Churchill Livingstone, Edinburgh, p. 65.

PETERS, T.G., DONEGAN, W.L. and BURG, E.A. (1979) Minimal breast cancer. A clinical appraisal. *Ann. Surg.*, **145**, 104.

PEYSTER, R.G. and KALISHER, L. (1979) Needle localization of non-palpable lesions of the breast. *Surg., Gynaecol. Obstet.*, **148**, 703–6.

PICKREN, J.W. (1961) Significance of occult metastases. A study of breast cancer. *Cancer*, **14**, 1266–71.

POCHACZEVSKY, R. and MEYERS, P.H. (1979) The value of vacuum contoured, liquid crystal, dynamic breast thermoangiography. *Acta thermogr.*, **4**, 8–16.

QUIMET-OLIVER, D. and HEBERT, G. (1974) Galactography: a method of detection of unsuspected cancers. *Am. J. Roentgenol.*, **120**, 55–61.

RAMSDEN, J.A., MOORES, B.M. and ASBURY, D.L. (1979) The dose to the patient and the quality of the image in xeromammography. *Br. J. Radiol.*, **52**, 804–9.

RASKIN, M.M., and MARTINEX-LOPEZ, M. (1976) Thermographic patterns of the breast; a critical analysis of interpretation. *Radiology*, **121**, 553–5.

REEVE, T.S., JELLINS, J., KOSSOFF, G. and BARRACLOUGH, B.H. (1978a) Ultrasonic visualization of breast cancer. *Aust. NZ. J. Surg.*, **48**, 278–81.

REEVE, T.S., JELLINS, J., KOSSOFF, G. and BARRACLOUGH, B.H. (1978b) in *Tumour Ultrasound* (eds C.R. Hill, V.R. McCready and D.O. Cosgrove). Pitman Medical, London, pp. 93–103.

RENWICK, S. (1976) The possible relationship between mammary dysplasia and breast cancer. *Aust. NZ. J. Surg.*, **46**, (4), 341–3.

REVESZ, G. (1978) Breast cancer screening: predictive values and strategies. *Acta thermogr.*, **3**, 150–4.

RIDOLFI, R.L., ROSEN, P.P., PORT, A., KINNE, D. and MIKE, V. (1979) Medullary carcinoma of the breast: a clinicopathological study with a 10-year follow-up. *Cancer*, **40**, 1365–85.

RIMSTEN, A., STENKVIST, B., JOHANSON, H. and LINDGREN, A. (1975) The diagnostic accuracy of palpation and fine needle biopsy and an evaluation of their combined use in the diagnosis of breast lesions. *Ann. Surg.*, **182**, 1.

RINI, J.M., HOROWITZ, A., BALTER, S. and WATSON, R.C. (1973) A comparison of tungsten and molybdenum as target material for mammographic X-ray tubes. *Radiology*, **106**, 657–61.

ROBERTS, J.G., PREECE, P.E., BOLTON, P.M., BAUM, M. and HUGHES, L.E. (1975) The 'tru-cut' biopsy in breast cancer. *Clin. Oncol.*, **1**, 297–303.

ROBBINS, G.F. (1962) Long-term survivals among primary operable breast cancer patients with metastatic axillary lymph nodes at level III. *Acta Un. Int. Cancer.*, **18**, 864–7.

ROGERS, L. and PAGE, D. (1979) Epithelial proliferative disease of the breast – a marker of increased cancer risk in certain age groups. *Dis. Breast*, **5**, (2), 2–7.

ROSATO, F.E., THOMAS, J. and ROSATO, E.F. (1973) Operative management of non-palpable lesions detected by mammography. *Surg. Gynaec. Obstet.*, **137**, 491–3.

ROSEN, P.P., SNYDER, R.E. and ROBBINS, G. (1974) Specimen radiography for non-palpable breast lesions found by mammography: procedures and results. *Cancer*, **34**, 2028–33.

ROSEN, P.P., LIEBERMAN, P.H., BRAUN, D.W., KOSLOFF, C. and ADAIR, F. (1978) Lobular carcinoma *in situ* of the breast. Detailed analysis of 99 patients with average follow-up of 24 years. *Am. J. Surg. Path.*, **2**, 225–51.

ROSES, D.F., HARRIS, M.N., GORSTEIN, F. and GUMPORT, S.L. (1980) Biopsy of microcalcification detected by mammography. *Surgery*, **87**, 248–52.

RUSS, J.E., WINCHESTER, D.P., SCANLON, E.F. and CHRIST, M.A. (1978) Cytological findings of aspiration of tumours of the breast. *Surg. Gynaecol. Obstet.*, **146**, 3, 407–11

SARTORIUS, O.W., MORRIS, P.L., BENEDICT, D.L. and SMITH, H.L. (1977) Contrast Ductography for recognition and localization of Benign and Malignant Breast Lesions; an improved technique in *Breast Carcinoma* (ed. W.W. Logan), John Wiley & Son, New York, pp. 281–300.

SCARFF, R.W. and TORLONI, H. (1968) Histological typing of breast tumours in *International Histological Classification of Tumours No. 2*, World Health Organisation, Geneva.

SCHNEIDER, R. (1970) Comparison of age, sex and incidence rates in human and canine breast cancer. *Cancer*, **26**, 419–26.

SCHWARTZ, G., PATCHEFSKY, A.S., FEIG, M.D., SHABER, G. and SCHWARTZ, A. (1980) Clinically occult breast cancer. *Ann. Surg.*, **191**, 8–12.

SEELENTAG, W.W. (1979) *Electrostatic X-ray imaging.* I.E.E. Medical Electronics Monographs, **28**, 1–64.

SELTZER, M.H., PERLOFF, L.J., KELLEY, R.I. and FITTIS, W.T. (1970) The significance of age in patients with nipple discharge. *Surg. Gynaecol. Obstet.*, **131**, 519–22.

SHABER, G.S., NERLINGER, R.E., FEIG, S.A., PATCHEFSKY, A.S. and SCHWARTZ, G.F. (1976) Thermography to detect breast cancer (letter). *New Engl. J. Med.*, **295**, 1082.

SHABOT, M.M., GOLDBERG, I.M., SCHICK, P. *et al.* (1982) Aspiration cytology is superior to tru-cut needle biopsy in establishing the diagnosis of clinically suspicious breast masses. *Ann. Surg.*, **196**, 122–6.

SHAPIRO, S., STRAX, P., VENET, L. and FINK, R. (1968) The search for risk factors in breast cancer. *Am. J. Public Health*, **58**, 820.

SHAPIRO, S. (1977) Evidence on screening for breast cancer from a randomized trial. *Cancer*, **39**, 2772–82.

SHAPIRO, S. (1976) *Decision making and Medical Care* (ed. F.T. De Dombal and F. Gremy), North-Holland Publishing Company, Amsterdam.

SICKLES, E.A. (1979) Microfocal spot magnification mammography using xero-radiographic and screen/film recording systems. *Radiology*, **131**, 599–607.

SICKLES, E.A., DOI, K. and GENANT, H.K. (1977) Magnification film mammography: image quality and clinical studies. *Radiology*, **125**, 69–76.

SICKLES, E.A. and GENANT, H.K. (1979) Controlled single blind clinical evaluation of low dose mammographic film/screen systems. *Radiology*, **130**, 347–51.

SILVERBERG, S.G., CHITAL, A.R., HIND, A.D., FRAZIER, A.B. and LEVITT, S.H. (1970) Sinus histiocytosis and mammary carcinoma: study of 366 radical mastectomies and an historical review. *Cancer*, **26**, 1177–85.

SIMON, N., LESNICK, G.J., LEVER, W.N. and BACHMAN, A.L. (1972) Roentgeno graphic localization of small lesions of the breast by the spot method. *Surg. Gynaec. Obstet.*, **134**, 572–4.

SIMON, N. and SILVERSTONE, S.M. (1976) Radiation as a cause of breast cancer. *Bull. NY Acad. Med.*, **52**, no 7.

STANTON, L., VILLAFANA, T., DAY, J.L., LIGHTFOOT, D.A. and STANTON, R.E. (1979) A study of mammographic exposures and detail visibility using three systems; Xerox 125, Min-R and Xonics XERG. *Radiology*, **132**, 455–62.

STARK, A.M. (1970) Screening for breast cancer. *Lancet*, ii, 407–9.

STARK, A.M. (1976) The significance of an abnormal breast thermogram. *Acta thermogr.*, **1**, 33–7.

STARK, A.M. and WAY, S. (1974) The use of thermovision in the detection of early breast cancer. *Cancer*, **33**, 1664–70.

STARK, A.M. and WAY, S. (1974) The screening of well women for the early detection of breast cancer using clinical examination with thermography and mammography. *Cancer*, **33**, 1671–9.

STEKETEE, J. (1973) Spectral emissivity of skin and pericardium. *Phys. Med. Biol.*, **18**, 686–94.

STEVELS, A.L.N. (1975) New phosphors for X-ray screens. *Medicamundi*, **20**, 12–22.

STEWART, F.W. and TREVES, N. (1948) Lymphangiosarcoma in post mastectomy lymphoedema. *Cancer*, **1**, 64.

STORM, E. and ISRAEL, H.I. (1970) Photon cross sections from 1 keV to 100 MeV for elements $Z = 1$ to $Z = 100$. *Nucl. Data Tables*, **7**, 565–688.

STRAX, P. (1980) Strategy (motivation) for detection of early breast cancer. *Cancer*, **46**, 926–9.

STRAX, P., VENET, L. and SHAPIRO, S. (1973) Value of mammography in reduction of mortality from breast cancer in mass screening. *Cancer*, **117**, 686–9.

SULLIVAN, J.J., MAGEE, H.R. and DONALD, K.J. (1977) Secretary (juvenile) carcinoma of the breast. *Pathology*. **9**, 341–6.

THOMAS, B. (1975) Selective screening for breast cancer in Guildford. *Lancet*, ii, 914–15.

THOMAS, J.M., FITZHARRIS, B.M., REDDING, W.H., WILLIAMS, J.E. *et al.* (1978) Clinical examination, xeromammography and fine needle aspiration cytology in the diagnosis of breast tumours. *Br. Med. J.*, **2**, 1139–41.

THREATT, B. and APPELMAN, H.D. (1973) Mammary duct injection. *Radiology*, **108**, 71–6.

TOKER, C. and GOLDBERG, J. (1977) Small cell lesion of mammary ducts and lobules. *Path. Ann.*, **1977**, 217–45.

TONEGUTTI, L.M., ACCIARRI, L. and RACANELLI (1980) Fundamentals of contact thermography in female breast diseases. *Acta thermogr.* Supp. 3.

TONGE, K., DAVIS, R. and MILLIS, R.R. (1976) The problem of discrimination in mammography. Arguments for using a biological test object. *Br. J. Radiol.*, **49**, 678–85.

TRICOIRE, J., MARIEL, L. and AMIEL, J.P. (1972) Thermographie en plaque et diagnostic des affections du sein. *J. Radiol. Electol. Med. Nucl.*, **53**, 13–16.

UICC (1974) *TNM Classification of Malignant Tumours*, 2nd edn (ed. M.H. Harmer), International Union against Cancer, Geneva.

UICC (1978) *TNM Classification of Malignant Tumours*, 3rd edn (ed. M.H. Harmer), International Union against Cancer, Geneva.

UICC (1980) *TNM Classification of Malignant Tumours: A Brochure of Check Lists* (ed. A.H. Sellers), International Union against Cancer, Geneva.

UICC (1980) *TNM Classification of Malignant Tumours*. UICC Technical Report Series, Vol. 51, Geneva.

UPTON, A.C., BEEBE, G.W., BROWN, J.M., QUIMBY, E.H. and SHELLABARGER, C. (1977) Report of NCI AdHoc Working Group on the risks associated with mammography in mass screening for the detection of breast cancer. *J. Natl. Cancer Inst.*, **59**, 480–93.

URBAN, J.A. (1977) Changing patterns of breast cancer. *Bull. NY Acad. Med.*, 749–53.

VAN BOGAERT, L.J. and MALDAGUE, P. (1978) Histologic classification of pure primary epithelial breast cancer. *Human Path.*, **9**, 175–80.

VAN DE RIET, W.G. and WOLFE, J.N. (1977) Dose reduction in xeroradiography of the breast. *Am. J. Roentgenol.*, **128**, 821–3.

VENET, L. (1980) Self examination and clinical examination of the breast. *Cancer*, **46**, 930–2.

VESSEY, M.P., MCPHERSON, K. and DOLL, R. (1981) Breast cancer and oral contraceptives: findings in Oxford-Family Planning Association contraceptive study. *Br. Med. J.*, **282**, 2093–4.

WAGNER, R.F. and WEAVER, K.E. (1976) Prospects for X-ray exposure reduction using rare-earth intensifying screens. *Radiology*, **118**, 183–8.

WEBB, J. (1975) A cytological study of mammary disease. *Ann. R. Coll. Surg.*, **56**, 181–91.

WEBSTER, E.W. and KALISHER, L. (1977) in *Breast Carcinoma: the Radiologist's Expanded Role* (ed. W.W. Logan), John Wiley and Sons Inc., New York, pp. 197–206.

WEISS, J.P. and WAYRYNEN, R.E. (1976) Imaging system for low dose mammography. *J. Appl. Photogr. Eng.*, **2**, 7–10.

WELLINGS, S.R., JENSEN, H.M. and MARCUM, R.G. (1975) An atlas of subgross pathology of the human breast with special reference to possible precancerous lesions. *J. Natl. Cancer Inst.*, **55**, 231–73.

WELLINGS, S.R. and WOLFE, J.N. (1978) Correlative study of the histological and radiographic appearances of the breast parenchyma. *Radiology*, **129**, 299–306.

WESTBROOK, K.C. and GALLAGER, H.S. (1975) Intraductal carcinoma of the breast. *Am. J. Surg.*, **130**, 667–70.

WHEELER, J.E. and ENTERLINE, H.T. (1976) in *Pathology Annual* (vol. II), (ed. S.C. Sommers), Appleton Century Crofts, New York, 161–88.

WHITBY, L.G. (1968) *Br. J. Hosp. Med.*, **1**, 79–91.

WHITE, L., CORNELIUS, J., JUDKINS, A. and PATTERSON, J. (1978) Screening of cancer by nurses. *Cancer Nurs.*, (February) 15–20.

WILSON, J.M.G. and JUNGNER, G. (1968) *Principles and Practice of Screening for Disease.* W.H.O., Geneva.

WOLFE, J.N. (1972) *Xeroradiography of the breast.* Charles C. Thomas, Springfield, Illinois.

WOLFE, J.N. (1974) Analysis of 462 breast carcinomas. *Am. J. Roentgenol.*, **121**, 846–53.

WOLFE, J.N. (1976a) Breast patterns as an index of risk for developing breast cancer. *Am. J. Roentgenol.*, **126**, 1130–9.

WOLFE, J.N. (1976b) Risk for breast cancer development determined by mammographic parenchymal pattern. *Cancer*, **37**, 2486–92.

WOLFE, J.N. (1977) Mammography a radiologist's view. *JAMA*, **237**, no. 20, 2223–4.

WOLFE, J.N. (1979) *Xeroradiography: uncalcified breast masses*, Charles C. Thomas, Springfield, Illinois.

WYNDER, E.L. (1969) Identification of women at high risk for breast cancer. *Cancer*, **24**, 1235–40.

XEROX CORPORATION (1974 onwards). *Tech. Applic. Bull.*, **1–9**.

ZAJICEK, J. (1979) *Diagnostic Cytology and its histopathologic bases*, 3rd edn, Lippinicott Co, Philadelphia, ch. 29.

ZAJDELA, A. (1975) The value of aspiration cytology in the diagnosis of breast cancer. Experience at the Foundation Curie. *Cancer*, **35**, 499.

ZEMAN, G.H., RAO, G.U.V. and OSTERMAN, F.A. (1976) Evaluation of xeroradiographic image quality. *Radiology*, **119**, 689–95.

ZISKIN, M.C., NEGIN, M., PINER, C. and LAPAYOWKER, M.S. (1975) Computer diagnosis of breast thermograms. *Radiology*, **115**, 341–7.

INDEX

Abscess, 42, 125
Acne, 139
Acute mastitis, 42, 125
Adenoid cystic carcinoma, 19
Adenoma, 24, 43
Adenoma of nipple, 43
Anode materials, 81
    and absorbed dose, 94
    and contrast, 93
Axillary lymph nodes
    accuracy of assessment, 187
    metastases, 183
    normal appearance, 183

Back-scatter, 79
Benign mammary dysplasia
    clinical features, 41
    histology, 22
    mammographic features, 101
Benign pairs, 209
Biopsy rate, 256, 262
Breast biopsy, 255
Breast carcinoma
    calcification, 161
    cytological features, 207
    histological classification, 8
    inflammatory, 152
    intracystic papillary, 158
    mammographic density, 144
    medullary, 158
    mucoid, 158
    outline, 154
    relative incidence, 8
Breast pain, 27

Calcification
    associated with a mass, 162
    in BMD, 106
    in comedo carcinoma, 168
    distribution, 162
    features in malignancy, 161
    number, 174
    shape, 168
    size, 168
Cancerization, 10
Carcinoids, 19
Clinical history, 250
Colloid carcinoma, 16
Compression in mammography, 77
Cyclical changes, 27
Cyclical mastalgia, 250
Cysts
    clinical features, 41
    cystography, 110
    differentiation from fibroadenoma, 110
    mamographic features, 109
    mural calcification, 110
Cystic hyperplasia, 22
Cystography, 158
Cystosarcoma phylloides, 21, 43, 130, 132
Cytology
    accuracy, 204, 210
    aspiration technique, 205
    in BMD, 210
    of cyst fluid, 210
    fat necrosis, 211
    features of benignancy, 207
    features of malignancy, 207
    of impalpable lesions, 206
    inflammatory lesions, 211
    medullary carcinoma, 209
    mucoid carcinoma, 209
    of nipple discharge, 204
    role, 203
    small cell carcinoma, 210

Diagnostic accuracy, 212
Diagnostic flowcharts, 245–247, 249
Disturbed architecture, 160
Duct abnormalities
    in BMD, 114
    ectasia, 23, 43, 119
    papilloma, 133
    in tumour, 160
Ductography, 197–200

Fat necrosis
    clinical features, 42
    histology, 24
    radiology, 134, 139
f-Factor, 79
Fibroadenoma
    calcification, 130
    clinical features, 43
    giant, 132
    histology, 24
    mammographic features, 125
Fibroadenosis
    clinical features, 40–41
    histology, 22
Fibrocystic disease, 22
Fibrous mastopathy, 42
Film receptors, 83–85, 94–95
    characteristic curve, 84
    contrast enhancement, 84
    energy absorption coefficient, 85
    film latitude, 84
    film sensitivity, 85
    resolution, 84
Film/screen receptors, 85–88, 95
    characteristic curve, 86
    contact, 86, 88
    contrast, 85
    film sensitivity, 88
    resolution, 85
    screen construction, 86
    screen sensitivity, 87
Filters, 81
Fine needle aspiration, 256
Foamy histiocytes, 210
Focal spot size, 92
Frank needle, 196
Frequency response, 92
Frozen section, 1

Galactocele, 42

Geometric unsharpness, 92
Grid mammograms, 99
Gynaecomastia, 43

Haematoma, 133
Half value layers, 82
Hamartoma, 24
Histological grading, 49
Host resistance, 20

Image contrast, 77, 82
Image sharpness, 77
Impalpable lesions
    biopsy technique, 200
    cytology, 206
    localization by coned views, 74
    need for localization, 192
    needle localization, 193
    specimen radiography, 192
Increased vascularity, 180
Infiltrating carcinoma
    prognostic factors, 20, 46
Infiltrating duct carcinoma
    associated in situ tumour, 13
    histology, 13
    histological grading, 14
    histological variants, 15
    nuclear grading, 15
Infiltrating lobular carcinoma
    histology, 17
Inflammatory carcinoma, 19
Infra-red photography, 221–222
Infra-red thermography, 214–234
    accuracy, 222, 225–227
    detector systems, 215
    equipment, 215
    future prospects, 233
    predictive value, 229
    preliminary cooling, 217
    in screening, 229–231
In situ carcinoma
    clinical features, 47
    definition, 9
    electron microscopy, 9
In situ duct carcinoma
    calcification, 10
    gross appearances, 5
    histological features, 9
    multifocal nature, 10
    recurrent, 10

In situ lobular carcinoma
  associated calcification, 12
  bilaterality, 12
  histology, 11
  incidence, 11
  multifocal nature, 12
  recurrent, 12
Intramammary lymph node, 44
Ionography, 99
Isotherms, 215–216

Lactational tumours, 48
Lebourgne's Law, 46, 154
Leukaemia, 21
Lipid secreting tumours, 19
Lipoma, 44, 133
Liquid crystal thermography, 214,
  232–233
Lobular carcinoma, 6
Lymph node assessment, 50
Lymph nodes
  axillary level, 7
Lymphoedema, 141
Lymphoma, 21

Magnification mammography, 98
Mammary fibrosis, 105
Mammographic views, 54–75
  axillary tail oblique, 67
  cranio-caudad, 61
  erect axillary, 70
  erect latero-medial, 59
  erect medio-lateral, 57
  extended cranio-caudad, 64
  oblique, 65
  for screening, 54
  selection of technique, 55
  supine axillary, 72
  supine medio-lateral, 56
Mammography, 101–191
  false negative, 254
  false positive, 254
  indications, 253
  predictive value, 229
  roles in cancer, 142
  signs of cancer, 144, 177
  sponges, 72
Mastectomy specimen
  pathological examination, 7

Medullary carcinoma
  cytology, 209
  gross appearance, 4
  histology, 15
  radiology, 158
Metachronous tumours, 53
Metaplasia, 19
Metastases to the breast, 21, 51
Metastatic staging, 51
Minimal breast cancer, 20
Modulation transfer function, 92
Mondor's disease, 36
Mucinous tumours, 19
Mucoid carcinoma
  cytology, 209
  histology, 16
  radiology, 158

Needle biopsy, 2
  Tru-cut, 2
Nipple abnormalities
  discharge, 28, 250
  Paget's disease, 38, 250
  retraction, 28, 36, 250
  ulceration, 28
Nipple discharge, 28, 197–199
  biopsy technique, 201
  cytology, 203

Oil cysts, 139

Paget's disease
  association with *in situ* cancer, 11
  clinical features, 38
  cytology, 204–205
  histology, 19
Pain, 250
Palpation, 38
Papillary carcinoma
  histology, 19
  radiology, 158
Papilloma
  clinical features, 43
  histology, 24
Papillomatosis
  histology, 23
  radiology, 114, 117
Parenchymal patterns, 187, 189–190
  and cancer incidence, 189
  and other risk factors, 190
  Wolfe classification, 189

Peau d'orange, 48
Performance criteria, 76
Physical examination, 32
Physical signs, 250
Plasma cell mastitis, 120
Preliminary biopsy, 2
Profile scanning, 216
Prognostic factors, 20, 48–51, 258

Quantum mottle, 87–88

Radiation
    dose, 79, 82, 95–96
    exposure, 78, 96
    hazard, 76, 254
Risk factors
    age, 29, 260
    BMD, 260
    family history, 31, 260
    hair dye, 261
    high fat diet, 261
    hormonal status, 260
    hormone manipulation, 30, 261
    nulliparity, 32
    previous benign disease, 31
    sex, 260
    smoking, 261

Sarcomas, 21, 52
Scarring, 139, 141
    calcification, 141
Scatter, 78
Scirrhous carcinoma
    gross appearances, 4
Sclerosing adenosis
    clinical features, 42
    histology, 23
    mammographic features, 106
Screening for breast cancer
    high risk groups, 260
    populations, 257–258
    results, 263
Secretory disease, 119
Sentinel cells, 208
Skin changes
    after radiotherapy, 179
    clinical features, 34, 41
    in inflammatory carcinoma, 152
    thickening, 177
Skin dimpling, 250

Skin emissivity, 214
Specimen radiography, 6
Squamous cell carcinoma, 19
Stefan's constant, 214
Symptomatology, 26

Thermal asymmetry, 227
Thermal patterns
    abnormal, 223
    classification, 219
    cyclical variation, 219
    diurnal variation, 219
    edge effect, 229
    mechanism of abnormality, 227–228
    normal, 218
    and oral contraceptives, 219
    in pregnancy, 219
Thermography, 255
    prognostic value, 255
TNM staging, 251–252

Ultrasound
    accuracy, 242–243, 245
    BMD, 242, 244
    clinical role, 246, 255
    cyst, 241, 244
    effect of age, 240
    equipment, 236
    fat necrosis, 244
    fibroadenoma, 242, 244
    infiltrating lesions, 243–244
    medullary carcinoma, 243–244
    normal, 239
    principles, 235
    resolution, 243

Venous diameter ratio, 227

Xeroradiography
    edge enhancement, 91, 98
    exposure latitude, 91
    latent image, 89
    negative mode, 90
    performance, 95
    positive mode, 90
    powder development, 90
    quantum mottle, 91
    radiation dose, 98
    selenium plate, 89
    125 System, 92
    sensitivity, 89

Xonics, 99
X-ray attenuation, 77
X-ray spectra, 81